In Clinical Practice

Taking a practical approach to clinical medicine, this series of smaller reference books is designed for the trainee physician, primary care physician, nurse practitioner and other general medical professionals to understand each topic covered. The coverage is comprehensive but concise and is designed to act as a primary reference tool for subjects across the field of medicine.

More information about this series at http://www.springer.com/series/13483

Andrew Severn
Editor

Cognitive Changes after Surgery in Clinical Practice

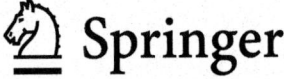 Springer

Editor
Andrew Severn
Department of Anaesthesia
Royal Lancaster Infirmary
Lancaster, Lancashire
United Kingdom

ISSN 2199-6652   ISSN 2199-6660   (electronic)
In Clinical Practice
ISBN 978-3-319-75722-3   ISBN 978-3-319-75723-0   (eBook)
https://doi.org/10.1007/978-3-319-75723-0

Library of Congress Control Number: 2018954074

This Springer imprint is published by the registered company Springer
Nature Switzerland AG
The registered company address is: Gewerbestrasse 11, 6330 Cham, Switzerland

I wish to dedicate this work to my 'Giants of Geriatrics' who will never see the finished article, but whose interest in me at all stages of my career has resulted in the project:

Brian Payne (1946–2012), consultant geriatrician in Norwich, took me on as a raw senior house officer in 1982 and, with good humour, tolerated my attempt to set up an intensive care unit on his ward before delivering me, as a more holistic doctor, to anaesthesia.

Jed Rowe (1954–2008), consultant geriatrician from Birmingham, whose pithy description of our landmark 2002 Age Anaesthesia Association gathering: 'this group is the antidote to those who think that anaesthetists are machine minders' became a mantra in developing the ethos of the Association.

Gwyn Seymour (1949–2016), professor in medicine for the elderly, Aberdeen, who was the link between the British Geriatrics Society and the profession of anaesthesia from his early days as a postgraduate and who, as president of the Age Anaesthesia Association, laid the foundation for a lasting collaboration.

Foreword

Cognitive dysfunction following anaesthesia for surgery is common. Anecdotally many patients complain of cognitive problems, either post-operative delirium (POD) or post-operative cognitive dysfunction or deficit (POCD) (or both), and some are wary of the implication of surgery for their later cognitive performance. It would appear that POD and POCD are unlikely to share the same pathophysiology: delirium is well defined with acute onset, whereas POCD has subtler effects with longer duration.[1] Other than a remote suggestion that post-traumatic stress disorder may be implicated, neither ICD11 nor DSM V mentions POCD as a separate diagnosis. This is surprising given the condition has been known about for many decades: a Lancet paper from 1955 expressly described adverse cerebral effects of anaesthesia in older patients, and subsequent research has identified this concern on many occasions.[2]

One of the difficulties of undertaking research on post-operative cognition is the multifactorial nature of the problem. Not only is it necessary to disaggregate delirium from longer-term cognitive dysfunction, but it is also essential to distinguish temporary from permanent effects. Many patients suffer short-term memory loss or difficulties in concentrating

---

[1]Krenk L, Rasmussen LS. Postoperative delirium and post-operative cognitive dysfunction in the elderly – what are the differences?" Minerva Anestesiol. 2011;77(7):742–9.
[2]Bedford PD. Adverse cerebral effects of anaesthesia on old people. Lancet. 1955;266(6884):259–64.

in the first 6 weeks to 3 months following surgery, and this usually attenuates with time. Some patients, however, seem to be permanently affected to varying degrees and show increasing signs of dementia; it is presently unclear if this is the result of the anaesthesia specifically or whether the disease was present preoperatively and is exacerbated or brought more to the fore as a result of surgery.

The value of this short book is in tackling many of these issues logically and comprehensively. POD and POCD are both consequences of surgery but, although related, must be considered separately. Dementia has now overtaken heart disease as the leading cause of death, and anything that can be done prophylactically is to be welcomed.[3] Understanding the specific techniques and drugs that may have implications for dementia is thus essential. However, regardless of preoperative cognitive status, general cognitive decline is important to patients and clinicians, and yet, the reasons for it is insufficiently known.

One of the critical issues for research in this area is having robust and replicable tools for assessing cognitive function. As in most areas of medicine, there has been a great deal of research over the years, but two problems always emerge: the relatively narrow focus of individual research papers and the lack of comparability because of differing assessment mechanisms used. Large differences are apparent in the literature including test batteries used, intervals between assessments, outcomes measured, statistical methods employed and the way in which neuropsychological deficits are defined.[4] Assessing cognitive function especially in dementia is important for decisions on when to intervene medically or socially, as well as in obtaining commensurate results for comparative analysis.

---

[3]Selbie D, Newton J. Health profile for England: telling a story about our health. Accessed on 7 Feb 2018 at https://publichealthmatters.blog.gov.uk/2017/07/13/health-profile-for-england-telling-a-story-about-our-health/.

[4]Rasmussen LS, Larsen K, Houx P, et al. The assessment of post-operative cognitive function. Acta Anaesthsiol Scand. 2001;45(3):275–89.

The type of surgery is also relevant to outcomes. Coronary artery surgery is especially problematic although other major surgical interventions lead to similar outcomes. Minimising the use of cardiopulmonary bypass during coronary artery bypass grafting may reduce cerebral micro-emboli, in itself a good outcome, but it does not reduce POCD at 1 week or 3 months.[5] In one study of noncardiac surgery, roughly 75% of patients showed no cognitive decline, whilst of those with cognitive deficits, half showed mild effects but 20% had severe decline (i.e. 5% overall).[6] In a separate paper, older people (over 60 years) were described as at significant risk for long-term cognitive problems (and worryingly patients with POCD at increased risk of death) in the first year after surgery. Independent risk factors for POCD at 3 months post-surgery were increasing age, lower educational attainment, a history of cerebrovascular accidents with no residual impairment and POCD at discharge.[7]

Alternative multifactorial strategies may be required, focussing not only on choice of anaesthetic drugs used but on post-operative recovery, such as sleep disturbance and environmental factors. Identifying inflammatory stress responses and multimodal **non-opioid** pain management may also assist.[8] However, research on dementia, notably on Alzheimer's disease, has thrown light on other factors, such as genetic features, in particular those related to apolipoprotein E genotype. Interestingly though, one recent paper suggests

[5]Liu YH, Wang DX, Li LH, et al. The effects of cardiopulmonary bypass on the number of cerebral micro-emboli and the incidence of cognitive dysfunction after coronary artery bypass graft surgery. Anesth Analg. 2009;109(4):1013–22.

[6]Price CC, Garvan CW, Monk TG. Type and severity of cognitive decline in older adults after non-cardiac surgery. Anesthesiology. 2008;108(1):8–17.

[7]Monk TG, Weldon BC, Garvan CW, et al. Predictors of cognitive dysfunction after major non-cardiac surgery. Anesthesiology. 2001;108(1):18–30.

[8]Krenk L, Rasmussen LS, Kehlet H. New insights into the pathophysiology of post-operative cognitive dysfunction. Acta Anaesthsiol Scand. 2010;54(8):951–6.

that the specific patterns of post-operative cognitive deficit were found to be independent of apolipoprotein E genotype and resembled vascular mild cognitive impairment.[9] This perhaps supports the conclusions of another research group that intraoperative monitoring of anaesthetic depth and cerebral oxygenation in noncardiac surgery might assist in reducing POCD, which they argue is probably more persistent than is currently understood.[10]

Overall, this book addresses a relatively neglected area. As the population ages and more people require surgery, it is vitally important that more information is obtained on what causes POCD and POD, how the occurrence of cognitive dysfunctions can be minimised, and what ways surgery and anaesthesia can be modified appropriately. Not least, this will be because clinicians are faced with increasing difficulties in dealing with patients whose ability to consent may be compromised. The papers in the book are intended to identify the latest best practice and to provide guidance for surgical teams in offering the best possible care. All involved will surely find valuable directions for future practice.

Lancaster, UK   Christopher Heginbotham

[9]Ancelin ML, de Roquefeuil G, Scali J, et al. Long-term post-operative cognitive decline in the elderly: the effects of anesthesiatype, apolipoprotein E genotype, and clinical antecedents. J Alzheimers Dis. 2010;22:S105–13.

[10]Ballard C, Jones E, Gauge N, et al. Optimised anaesthesia to reduce post-operative cognitive decline (POCD) in older patients undergoing elective surgery, a randomised controlled trial. PLoS One. 2012;7(6):e37410.

Preface

This book has evolved since the publishers approached me in 2015. Initially, I thought that a 'state of the science' on all matters pertaining to cognitive dysfunction in surgical patients could be drawn into a single volume. In my enthusiasm for the project, I had ignored the fact that many of the world's leading scientists and clinicians were publishing their own data without the need to involve me. What has developed is very different from that originally envisaged, but probably better.

This book celebrates the cooperation of clinicians and laypeople that occurs in a well-functioning hospital. Its authors are very much involved in the day-to-day management of frail elderly patients on surgical wards, and the format, subject matter, and length should make this a valuable adjunct to the ward library.

Lancaster, UK   Andrew Severn
March 2018

Contents

About the Authors

Gemma Alcorn, MBChB, MRCP is a senior registrar in geriatric medicine and general internal medicine in Southeast Scotland. Her specialist interests include management of frail elderly patients in the perioperative period and prevention of inappropriate admissions to secondary care. She is currently completing a Master's degree by research at the University of Edinburgh investigating the factors influencing acute admissions to hospital from care homes and is a clinical tutor at the University of Edinburgh Medical School.

Stephen Alcorn, MA, MRCP, FRCA is a senior registrar in anaesthesia in Southeast Scotland who completed his undergraduate studies at the University of Oxford and has undertaken postgraduate training in anaesthesia in Scotland and South Africa. He has a specialist interest in perioperative medicine and safe delivery of anaesthesia for older patients, in particular those with cognitive dysfunction. He has previously published on a variety of topics linked to anaesthesia including a review of perioperative management of patients with dementia.

Tamas Bakoyni, MD, EDIC qualified in medicine at the University Pécs, Hungary. He trained in anaesthesia and intensive care medicine in Hungary before moving to work in the UK where he developed an interest in long-term outcomes from critical illness. He is currently a senior clinical fellow in critical care at Imperial College NHS Trust, London.

Daniele Bryden, LLB, MML, FRCA, FFICM has been a consultant in intensive care medicine and anaesthesia in Sheffield since 2001. She has a background in training and examinations. She was lead examiner for the critical care component of the MRCS, national critical care tutor for the Royal College of Surgeons, and examiner for the Faculty of Intensive Care Medicine. Her clinical and research interests are focussed on decision-making and frailty assessment in critical care.

She has edited four medical textbooks and written a number of book chapters and review articles on aspects of professional practice and decision-making and is an editor of BJA Education. She also works as an associate professional assessor for the GMC and in 2013 was awarded the Pinkerton Medal by the Association of Anaesthetists of Great Britain and Ireland.

Christopher Heginbotham, MSc, MA, MPhil, PhD, FRSPH worked as chief executive of a number of NHS Trusts and health authorities as well as at Mind, the National Association for Mental Health. He is now emeritus professor of Mental Health Policy at the University of Central Lancashire. During the 1980s, he was successively a member of Hampstead Health Authority and Redbridge and Waltham Forest DHA and subsequently chairman of Redbridge and Waltham Forest FHSA. In 2008, he was appointed as a non-executive director of Lancashire Care Foundation Trust, a position he held until 2014. A physicist by background, he later trained in health-care ethics and epidemiology. His recent books, written with Dr Karen Newbigging, are *Commissioning Health and Wellbeing* (2014) and a four volume compendium on public health (2016), both for Sage.

Andrew Larner, MD, PhD, MRCP is a consultant neurologist at the Cognitive Function Clinic, Walton Centre for Neurology and Neurosurgery, Liverpool, UK. He is the author of *Neuropsychological Neurology: The Neurocognitive Impairments of Neurological Disorders* (Cambridge University Press 2013) and *Transient Global Amnesia: From Patient Encounter to Clinical Neuroscience* (Springer 2017) and has edited a multi-author volume entitled *Cognitive Screening Instruments: A Practical Approach* (Springer 2017).

Shane O'Hanlon, LLB, MRCPI is a consultant physician in geriatric and general internal medicine at St Vincent's University Hospital, Dublin. He holds an adjunct post as assistant professor at University College Dublin. He trained in surgical liaison geriatrics, working on surgical wards at the Royal Berkshire NHS Foundation Trust to provide perioperative care for older people. He has a particular interest in measures to identify and reduce post-operative delirium. He has been an invited speaker at several national and international meetings, including the Association of Anaesthetists of Great Britain and Ireland (AAGBI) Annual Congress, Proactive Care of Older People Undergoing Surgery (POPS), European Association of Urology and the Dingle Perioperative Conference. He is the honorary secretary of the British Geriatrics Society.

Valerie Page, FRCA, FFICM trained in Manchester and is a consultant in anaesthesia and critical care at Watford General Hospital. She is the UK clinical leader in ICU delirium and a hands-on clinical trialist having been the chief investigator on two interventional delirium randomised controlled trials in mechanically ventilated patients at Watford General Hospital. She is a key member of the international initiative to develop core outcome sets (COS) for delirium research. She is the author of a number of original research papers, reviews, editorials and clinical handbook *Delirium in Critical Illness*, currently in its 2nd edition (Cambridge Medicine 2015). Dr Page is a committee member of the European Delirium Association and an honorary senior clinical lecturer at Imperial College and the University of Hertfordshire.

Gary Rycroft, LLB (Vic) read law at the University of Manchester 1991–1994 and has a postgraduate diploma in legal practice at the College of Law (now University of Law) at Chester 1994–1995. He was admitted to the Roll of Solicitors in 1998. Throughout his career, Gary has specialised in private client law: wills, trusts, probate, will disputes and mental capacity. He is the senior partner at Joseph A. Jones & Co LLP in Lancaster. He sits on the National Mental Capacity Forum Leadership Group and is chair of the Dying Matters Forum (part of the charity Hospice UK).

Gary is the author of the chapter "Charities as Beneficiaries" for the Lexis Nexis publication *Administration of Estates* and lectures and writes regularly about the Mental Capacity Act and advance care planning. On television, he is the resident legal expert on the BBC1 consumer affairs programme *Rip Off Britain* and regularly appears on the radio and in print media.

Andrew Severn, FRCA is a consultant anaesthetist from Lancaster. He has been involved in curriculum development for the Royal College of Anaesthetists in respect of perioperative management of elderly patients, being a commissioning editor for the College's e-learning programme from 2007 to 2009. He was a council member of the Age Anaesthesia Association from 2000 to 2011 and organised three of its annual meetings. He published a 1988 *British Journal of Anaesthesia* review on parkinsonism and a number of chapters in textbooks of geriatric medicine and specialist textbooks about geriatric anaesthesia. Recently semi-retired, Andrew teaches physiology and supervises problem-based learning at Lancaster Medical School.

Chapter 1
Dementia and the Health of the Nation

Andrew Larner

Introduction: The Scale of the Dementia Challenge

It is said that when Dr Alois Alzheimer made his presentation entitled "On a peculiar disease process of the cerebral cortex", in which the clinical and neuropathological findings in his patient, Auguste D., were first delivered [1], the audience at the 37th Conference of the South-West German Psychiatrists in Tübingen on that November day in 1906 made no comments and asked no questions. Even following Alzheimer's eponymous immortalization by Emil Kraepelin in the 8th edition of the latter's psychiatry textbook published in 1910, and the publication of the first cases in the English language in 1912 by Solomon Carter Fuller [2], "Alzheimer's disease" (AD) continued to be viewed as a very rare presenile form of dementia. Indeed, it was not until the equation of "senile dementia" with "Alzheimer's disease" in the 1960s and 1970s, based on the work of Tomlinson and

A. Larner
Cognitive Function Clinic, Walton Centre for Neurology
and Neurosurgery, Liverpool, UK
e-mail: a.larner@thewaltoncentre.nhs.uk

© Springer International Publishing AG, part of Springer Nature 2018
A. Severn (ed.), *Cognitive Changes after Surgery in Clinical Practice*, In Clinical Practice,
https://doi.org/10.1007/978-3-319-75723-0_1

Roth in the United Kingdom [3] and Robert Katzman in the Unites States of America [4], that the prevalence, morbidity and mortality of this condition was realised, transforming AD from a rare eponymous condition to an issue of major social, economic, and political significance [5].

As increasing age is recognised to be the major (unmodifiable) risk factor for the development of AD and other neurodegenerative forms of dementia, it is immediately obvious that the prevalence of dementia will increase as the population ages. Much research effort has been expended in recent years in epidemiological studies of dementia prevalence and incidence, especially of AD. The large majority of these investigations have indicated an increasing burden of disease, with patient numbers predicted to increase dramatically worldwide in the coming decades [6–8]. Alongside the human cost, to both patients and their carers, these numbers will have significant societal and financial cost implications [7, 9]. For example, a 2010 global cost of illness study suggested a "base case option" figure of US$604 billion, equivalent to the 18th largest national economy in the world (between Turkey and Indonesia), and larger than the revenue of the world's largest companies (Wal-Mart, Exxon Mobil) at that time. In high income countries, which accounted for 89% of the costs but only 46% of dementia prevalence, this was mostly due to the direct costs of social care, whilst in low and middle income countries, which accounted for only 11% of the costs but 54% of dementia prevalence, this was mostly due to informal care costs [9]. Such figures indicate the need to take action now, if possible, the moreso if one factors into this consideration the likelihood that many dementia cases remain undetected in the community (meta-analytic pooled rate of undetected dementia in 23 suitable studies was a staggering 61.7%) [10].

This grim epidemiological picture is compounded by the current absence of effective treatments for dementia. Although cholinesterase inhibitors (donepezil, rivastigmine, and galantamine) and memantine are licensed for the symptomatic treatment of AD in many countries, their effects are variable and at best modest, with no evidence for a disease modifying effect. Experimental pharmacotherapies, many developed on the basis of the predictions of the amyloid hypothesis of AD pathogenesis, have failed to translate to the clinical arena, despite initially encouraging findings in animal models of AD.

Although the possible discovery of effective disease modifying treatments for dementia cannot be ruled out, it seems unlikely that the traditional, "reactive", model of disease management – in which patients present with symptoms which doctors evaluate, diagnose, and treat – will suffice in this context. Something more proactive is going to be required in the future: at the current time it seems likely that preventative measures constitute a more viable approach. Certainly this has been an increasing subject of interest to dementia researchers in recent years [11, 12]. Such preventative measures will require a significant change in the approach to medical management, also encompassing political action.

Dementia Has Predementia and Preclinical Phases

In this context, it is worth remembering that dementia is a disease process rather than an event (with perhaps the exception of the very rare instances of "strategic infarct dementia" affecting cognitively eloquent structures). For example, in the case of AD it is evident from longitudinal studies of individuals harbouring deterministic mutations for early-onset disease that changes are occurring in the brain for many years prior to the onset of the clinical symptoms of cognitive change [13, 14]. The presymptomatic or preclinical phase is succeeded by a predementia or prodromal phase (nomenclature of Dubois et al. [15]); the latter has previously been characterised as "mild cognitive impairment" (MCI), and further categorised according to the neuropsychological phenotype as amnestic MCI, single non-memory domain MCI, or multiple domain MCI. However, some authorities prefer to diagnose "prodromal AD" or

TABLE I.I   Biomarkers of AD at any disease stage

Diagnostic markers (specific for presence of amyloid or tau pathology):
Cerebrospinal fluid:
    Reduced Abeta1–42
    Raised total-tau protein or phospho-tau protein
Amyloid Positron Emission Tomography (amyloid PET):
    Deposition of Abeta1-42
[In development: *Tau Positron Emission Tomography (tau PET):*
    Deposition of tau protein]
Progression markers (downstream markers, lacking pathological specificity):
Fluorodeoxyglucose Positron Emission Tomography (FDG PET):
    Cortical hypometabolism, especially temporoparietal distribution.
Magnetic Resonance (MR) imaging:
    Atrophy of medial temporal cortex and hippocampus

early AD when possible, based on changes in disease 'biomarkers' that can be identified radiologically or biochemically (see Table 1.1) and which are now incorporated into diagnostic criteria for AD [16].

Other dementing disorders also have a symptomatic but predementia phase (e.g. MCI in Parkinson's disease dementia/dementia with Lewy bodies, vascular dementia, frontotemporal dementia [17–19]) and presymptomatic or preclinical phases. Hence there is a window of opportunity, lasting potentially decades, when interventions might slow or halt the pathogenetic processes, thereby delaying or preventing the clinical features of dementia.

Prevention: Individual Risk Prediction

Accurate, individually tailored, prediction of AD diagnosis cannot currently be made, with the exception of relatively rare individuals with a family history of early-onset AD with

TABLE 1.2 Genetic factors in AD

Early-onset familial AD
Autosomal dominant disease, deterministic mutations in genes coding for:
Amyloid precursor protein (APP)
Presenilin 1 (PSEN1)
Presenilin 2 (PSEN2)

an inheritance pattern in keeping with an autosomal dominant disorder. Mutations in three genes have been shown to be deterministic for early-onset familial AD (Table 1.2), namely amyloid precursor protein (APP), and presenilin 1 and 2 (PSEN1, PSEN2). If a pathogenic mutation can be defined in one or more affected family members, genetic counselling and predictive testing (in that order), using a model first developed in Huntington's disease, may be undertaken in at-risk individuals ("asymptomatic-at-risk AD" [15]). A similar approach may be taken in familial frontotemporal dementia. It should be emphasized that such cases constitute only a small proportion of all dementia, and moreover that there is at this time no effective disease modifying treatment that can be recommended to an individual with a predictive dementia diagnosis. The grim prospect of the future inevitability of disease may understandably discourage some at-risk individuals from accessing predictive testing.

In addition to deterministic genetic mutations, a number of genetic predisposing factors, of themselves neither necessary nor sufficient to cause AD, have been identified. Of these, the best known relates to apolipoprotein E (ApoE) genotypes, one of which (epsilon 4) increases AD risk, whereas another (epsilon 2) reduces it. The use of genome wide association screens (GWAS) examining many thousands of patients and controls has broadened the number of identified possible genetic risk factors for AD [20, 21].

GWAS studies have produced large datasets which allow genetic information to be matched with clinical and laboratory information and from which an epidemiological framework for individual risk prediction can be constructed. For example, a recent study [21] constructed a "polygenic hazard score" (PHS) for late-onset AD, the most common form of the disease, which incorporated 33 single nucleotide polymorphisms (SNPs) reported to increase the genetic risk of AD in case-control studies, including two variants of the ApoE gene. The PHS successfully stratified individuals into different risk strata in replication studies undertaken in independent patient samples. The age of AD onset predicted by the model was strongly associated with the actual age of onset. Likewise, PHS also strongly predicted time to progression to neuropathologically defined AD. Individual genetic profile and age could be translated into incidence rates, with PHS-predicted incidence strongly associated with empirical progression rates. In other words, individual differences in risk of developing AD could be quantified as a function of patient genotype and age. PHS was significantly associated with decreased CSF Abeta1–42 and increased CSF total-tau; and with greater neuroradiological volume loss in the medial temporal lobes [22].

The implications of this PHS, or any future instrument generated by similar means, are many [22, 23]. It may be used to estimate individual differences in AD risk across a patient's lifetime and to quantify the yearly incidence rate for developing AD. Such information might potentially be used at the individual level for the purpose of future planning, and at the collaborative level to enrich patient cohorts entering prevention and therapeutic trials (previous clinical trials may have failed, at least in part, because of inclusion of age-matched controls who were at high risk of progression to disease).

The approach used in this study is illustrative of an emerging trend, namely the development of "bioprediction" of brain disorder. This represents a reorientation of the medical concept of "disorder" which rejects the old binary or categorical formulation (disorder/normalcy) in favour of a probabilistic model based on present and future risks of harm. Such an approach is justified in part by the belief that disease biomarkers will not map cleanly onto clinical diagnostic categories. Matthew Baum has explored the bioethical issues, and has proposed a "probability dysfunction" model in which disorders are conceptualised as graphs of probability over time, the area under which would help to separate out self-limiting disorders from those with low probabilities of harm over longer time periods. "Risk banding", based on the shape of the probability function, is the strategy advocated to determine the necessity or otherwise for response/intervention [24]. PHS may be seen as a probability function which might be used to address individual risk of developing AD [23].

Prevention: Population Screening

The highly sophisticated methods required for genotyping and risk prediction may prove difficult to scale up to the population level, even though costs of genetic testing have fallen significantly in recent years. Hence, other strategies for the identification of individuals either in the early stages or at risk of dementia, and hence candidates for any identified disease modifying intervention, require exploration. To prevent dementia requires some form of screening process. How this might be effected requires careful consideration.

The classic criteria for disease screening were published under the auspices of the World Health Organisation (WHO) nearly 50 years ago (see Table 1.3) [25]. Guidelines and criteria for developing screening programmes have also been issued, such as those from the UK National Screening Committee (https://www.gov.uk/government/groups/uk-national-screening-committee-uk-nsc).

Of these conditions, some are fulfilled for dementia, such as the importance to public health with significant economic cost implications [5–9]. It is also clear that the natural history of most forms of dementia encompasses a presymptomatic/preclinical phase, with disease evolution occurring over many years before clinical presentation [13, 14, 17–19]. However, many other screening criteria are not (yet) fulfilled for dementia. None of the available pharmacotherapies for AD have been shown to be more beneficial when applied at the presymptomatic/preclinical stage compared to the later

TABLE 1.3 WHO screening criteria

The disease/condition sought should be an important public
health problem.

There should be a recognisable latent or presymptomatic stage
of the disease.

The natural history of the disease should be adequately
understood.

There should be a treatment for the condition, which should
be more beneficial when applied at the presymptomatic stage
compared to the later symptomatic stage.

There should be a suitable test or examination to detect the
disease with reasonable sensitivity and specificity.

The test should be acceptable to the population.

The healthcare system should have the capacity and policies in
place to test for the condition and deal with the consequences.

The cost of case finding, including diagnosis and treatment of
patients diagnosed, should be economically balanced in relation
to possible expenditure on medical care as a whole.

Case finding should be a continuing process and not a "once
and for all" project.

symptomatic stages. It is not clear whether healthcare sys-
tems have the capacity and policies to test for dementia and
deal with the consequences, nor that the cost of case finding,
including diagnosis and treatment, would be economically
balanced in relation to possible expenditure on medical care
as a whole [26].

Hesitation about the initiation of population screening,
particularly in the absence of a test or examination to detect
disease with reasonable sensitivity and specificity (with the
risk of large numbers of either false positive or false negative
diagnoses), is understandable [27, 28]. There are many existing cognitive screening instruments [29]. Initially these were
pen and paper tests but now are increasingly available as
online instruments, including web-based apps, which might
even be used in the future for patient self-assessment.
However, the many shortcomings of such cognitive screening instruments are well-recognised, not least that tests
which are too sensitive will identify many false positives

whilst tests which are too specific risk false negative diagnoses, both of which have a cost (emotional and financial). Furthermore, whether these screening instruments can reduce the acknowledged "dementia diagnosis gap", the difference between numbers of observed and expected cases of dementia (perhaps 50% in the UK [30]), let alone those at-risk of dementia, remains to be shown [31].

Dementia and Cognitive Impairment in the Surgical Population

A number of risk factors for AD have been identified which might form the basis for effective screening and possible intervention in populations presenting for surgery. These include vascular risk factors, such as midlife hypertension and hypercholesterolaemia, and diabetes mellitus. These vascular risk factors suggest possible cerebrovascular components in AD pathogenesis, and indeed there is neuropathological evidence of overlap between AD and vascular dementia, indicating that these changes most usually lie on a continuum or spectrum rather than representing "pure" conditions [32]. Amyloid PET imaging, an AD biomarker, shows amyloid deposition is associated strongly with traditional cardiovascular risk factors [33]. Such findings raise the possibility of modifiable risk factors for dementia (AD and vascular) which may be addressed, as for cardiovascular disease, even at the primary care level. Risk scores for prediction of dementia have been previously constructed, based on recognised mid-life vascular risk factors such as hypertension and hypercholesterolaemia (Fig. 1.1) [34].

In addition to these risk factors, it has been questioned whether the stress response of surgery may affect long term cognitive function. Post-operative delirium has been associated with more rapid cognitive decline, and more severe delirium with a greater rate of cognitive decline [35]. Surgery may also "unmask" pre-existing but clinically undeclared neurodegenerative disease giving the impression of "acute onset" [36].

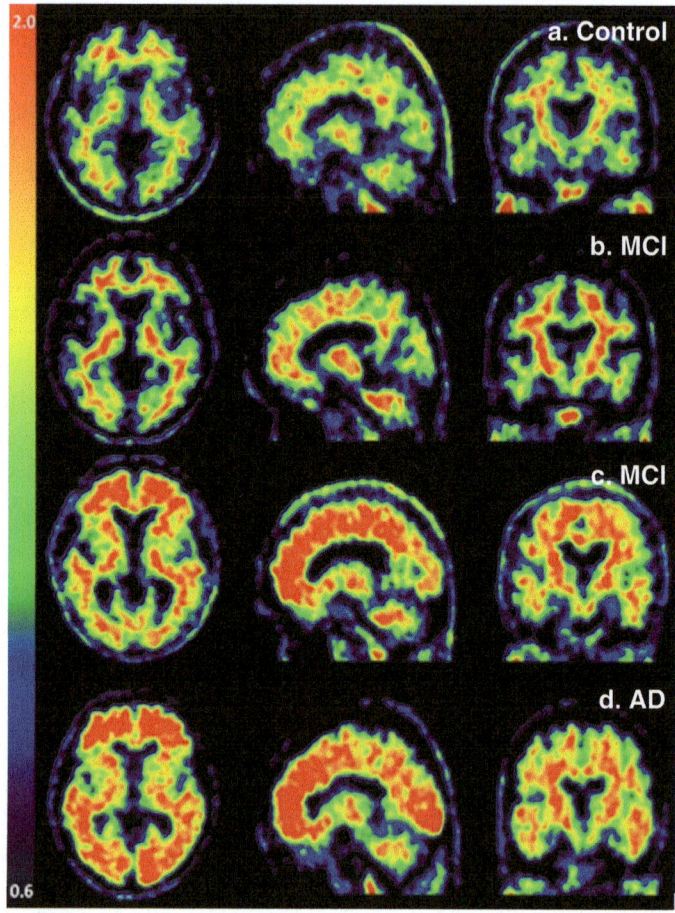

FIGURE 1.1 Amyloid (18F florbetapir) PET imaging, showing from left to right axial, sagittal and coronal brain images. Negative scans in a normal control subject (**a**) and a mild cognitive impairment (MCI) patient (**b**); positive scans in another MCI patient (**c**) and a patient with Alzheimer's disease (**d**). (Reproduced with permission from Eur J Nucl Med Mol Imaging. 2012 Apr;39(4):621–31. doi: 10.1007/s00259-011-2021-8. Epub 2012 Jan 18.)

The UK National Institute for Health and Care Excellence (NICE) issued a guideline in October 2015 whose title suggested a focus on dementia prevention, with recommendations aimed at the promotion of a healthy lifestyle, e.g. stop smoking, be more physically active, reduce alcohol consumption, adopt a healthy diet, and achieve and/or maintain a healthy weight [37]. There is some preliminary evidence of falling overall prevalence and incidence of dementia in the UK [38, 39]. Whether this reduction is a consequence of improved prevention and treatment of vascular risk factors, or due to other factors (e.g. better education, living conditions) is currently unknown [39]. Further longitudinal epidemiological studies may be required to answer such questions, but these are time-consuming and expensive. Pending definitive answers, it would not seem unreasonable to promote such interventions as likely preservers of brain health [40, 41]. It is argued that such "upstream primary prevention" has the largest effect on reduction of later dementia occurrence and disability [39].

Conclusion

The anticipated increase in the numbers of individuals with dementia as the world population ages threatens to overwhelm existing health and social care services. Interventions applied now which might contribute to the prevention of this eventuality should be welcomed. However, no intervention has yet been conclusively proven to reduce dementia risk at the individual or population level. Nevertheless, the identification of modifiable risk factors, such as midlife hypertension, hypercholesterolaemia, and diabetes mellitus, suggests that a vigorous screening policy to tackle these issues might pay long term dividends. Targeting individuals falling within a high risk band of a probability function, based on age and genotype, might ensure cost effective intervention.

Public health problems require public health solutions, which require political as well as clinical resolve and action. To this end, it is heartening to see initiatives to address these problems sponsored by the UK government, some with prime ministerial imprimatur [42–44], and by the international community (G8 nations) [45], even if these are by nature aspirational and relatively uncosted. It will require long-term commitment and funding from many sources to ensure the optimum management of dementia and to guarantee the brain health of all populations.

Acknowledgement   Thanks to Dr. Lauren Fratalia for critical comments on this manuscript.

References

1. Alzheimer A. Über eine eigenartige Erkrankung der Hirnrinde. Allgemeine Zeitschrift fur Psychiatrie und Psychisch-Gerichtlich Medizine. 1907;64:146–8.
2. Fuller SC. Alzheimer's disease (senium praecox): the report of a case and review of published cases. J Nerv Ment Dis. 1912;39:440–455 and 536–557.
3. Blessed G, Tomlinson BE, Roth M. The association between quantitative measures of dementia and of senile change in the cerebral grey matter of elderly subjects. Br J Psychiatry. 1968;114:797–811.
4. Katzman R. Editorial: the prevalence and malignancy of Alzheimer disease. A major killer. Arch Neurol. 1976;33:217–8.
5. World Health Organization. *Dementia: a public health priority*. Geneva: World Health Organization; 2012.
6. Ferri CP, Prince M, Brayne C, et al. Global prevalence of dementia: a Delphi consensus study. Lancet. 2005;366:2112–7.
7. Alzheimer's Society, *Dementia UK. A report into the prevalence and cost of dementia prepared by the Personal Social Services Research Unit (PSSRU) at the London School of Economics and the Institute of Psychiatry at King's College London, for the Alzheimer's Society*. London: Alzheimer's Society; 2007.
8. Prince M, Bryce R, Albanese E, Wimo A, Ribeiro W, Ferri CP. The global prevalence of dementia: a systematic review and metaanalysis. Alzheimers Dement. 2013;9:63–75.e2.
9. Prince M, Wimo A, Guerchet M, et al. *World Alzheimer report 2015. The global impact of dementia. An analysis of prevalence, incidence, cost and trends*. London: Alzheimer's Disease International; 2015.
10. Lang L, Clifford A, Wei L, et al. Prevalence and determinants of undetected dementia in the community: a systematic literature review and a meta-analysis. BMJ Open. 2017;7(2):e011146.

11. Prince M, Albanese E, Guerchet M, Prina M. *World Alzheimer report 2014. Dementia and risk reduction. An analysis of protective and modifiable factors.* London: Alzheimer's Disease International; 2014.

12. Kostoff RN, Zhang Y, Ma J, Porter AL, Buchtel HA. Prevention and reversal of Alzheimer's Disease: Georgia Institute of Technology; 2017. PDF. https://smartech.gatech.edu/handle/1853/56646.

13. Amieva H, Jacqmin-Gadda H, Orgogozo JM, et al. The 9 year cognitive decline before dementia of the Alzheimer type: a prospective population-based study. Brain. 2005;128:1093–101.

14. Jack CR Jr, Knopman DS, Jagust WJ, et al. Tracking pathophysiological processes in Alzheimer's disease: an updated hypothetical model of dynamic biomarkers. Lancet Neurol. 2013;12:207–16.

15. Dubois B, Feldman HH, Jacova C, et al. Revising the definition of Alzheimer's disease: a new lexicon. Lancet Neurol. 2010;9:1118–27.

16. Dubois B, Feldman HH, Jacova C, et al. Advancing research diagnostic criteria for Alzheimer's disease: the IWG-2 criteria. Lancet Neurol. 2014;13:614–29 [Erratum Lancet Neurol 2014;13:757].

17. Litvan I, Goldman JG, Troster AI, et al. Diagnostic criteria for mild cognitive impairment in Parkinson's disease: Movement Disorder Society task force guidelines. Mov Disord. 2012;27:349–56.

18. Gorelick PB, Scuteri A, Black SE, et al. Vascular contributions to cognitive impairment and dementia: a statement for healthcare professionals from the American Heart Association/American Stroke Association. Stroke. 2011;42:2672–713.

19. de Mendonça A, Ribeiro F, Guerreiro M, Garcia C. Frontotemporal mild cognitive impairment. J Alzheimers Dis. 2004;6:1–9.

20. Bertram L, Tanzi RE. Genome-wide association studies in Alzheimer's disease. Hum Mol Genet. 2009;18:R137–45.

21. Cuyvers E, Sleegers K. Genetic variations underlying Alzheimer's disease: evidence from genome-wide association studies and beyond. Lancet Neurol. 2016;15:857–68.

22. Desikan RS, Fan CC, Wang Y, et al. Genetic assessment of age-associated Alzheimer disease risk: development and validation of a polygenic hazard score. PLoS Med. 2017;14(3):e1002258. https://doi.org/10.1371/journal.pmed.1002258.

23. Larner AJ, Bracewell RM. Predicting Alzheimer's disease: a polygenic hazard score. J R Coll Physicians Edinb. 2017;47:151–2.
24. Baum ML. *The neuroethics of biomarkers. What the development of bioprediction means for moral responsibility, justice, and the nature of mental disorder.* Oxford: Oxford University Press; 2016.
25. Wilson JMG, Jungner G. Principles and practice of screening for disease. Public health paper no. 34. Geneva: World Health Organisation; 1968.
26. Larner AJ. Introduction to cognitive screening instruments: rationale and desiderata. In: Larner AJ, editor. Cognitive screening instruments. A practical approach. 2nd ed. London: Springer; 2017. p. 3–13.
27. Brunet MD, McCartney H, Heath I, et al. There is no evidence base for proposed dementia screening. BMJ. 2012;345:e8588.
28. Philips E, Walters A, Biju M, Kuruvilla T. Population-based screening for dementia: controversy and current status. Prog Neurol Psychiatry. 2016;20(1):6–9.
29. Larner AJ, editor. Cognitive screening instruments. A practical approach. 2nd ed. London: Springer; 2017.
30. Alzheimer's Society. *Mapping the Dementia Gap. Progress on improving diagnosis of dementia 2011–2012.* London: Alzheimer's Society; 2012. p. 2013.
31. Cagliarini AM, Price HL, Livemore ST, Larner AJ. Will use of the Six-Item Cognitive Impairment Test help to close the dementia diagnosis gap? Aging Health. 2013;9:563–6.
32. Schneider JA, Aggarwal NT, Barnes L, Boyle P, Bennett DA. The neuropathology of older persons with and without dementia from community versus clinic cohorts. J Alzheimers Dis. 2009;18:691–701.
33. Gottesman RF, Schneider AL, Zhou Y, et al. Association between midlife vascular risk factors and estimated brain amyloid deposition. JAMA. 2017;317:1443–50.
34. Kivipelto M, Ngandu T, Laatikainen T, Winblad B, Soininen H, Tuomilehto J. Risk score for the prediction of dementia in 20 years among middle aged people: a longitudinal, population-based study. Lancet Neurol. 2006;5:735–41.
35. Vasunilashorn SM, Fong TG, Albuquerque A, et al. Delirium severity post-surgery and its relationship with long-term cognitive decline in a cohort of patients without dementia. J Alzheimers Dis. 2017;61:347–58.

36. Larner AJ. "Dementia unmasked": atypical, acute aphasic, presentations of neurodegenerative dementing disease. Clin Neurol Neurosurg. 2005;108:8–10.
37. National Institute for Health and Care Excellence. Dementia, disability and frailty in later life – mid-life approaches to delay or prevent onset. London: NICE; 2015. NICE guidelines [NG16]. https://www.nice.org.uk/guidance/ng16
38. Matthews FE, Stephan BC, Robinson L, et al. A two decade dementia incidence comparison from the cognitive function and ageing studies I and II. Nat Commun. 2016;7:11398.
39. Wu YT, Fratiglioni L, Matthews FE, et al. Dementia in western Europe: epidemiological evidence and implications for policy making. Lancet Neurol. 2016;15:116–24.
40. Bennett DA. Banking against Alzheimer's. Sci Am Mind. 2016;27(4):28–37.
41. Northey JM, Cherbuin N, Pumpa KL, Smee DJ, Rattray B. Exercise interventions for cognitive function in adults older than 50: a systematic review with meta-analysis. Br J Sports Med. 2018;52:154–60.
42. Department of Health. Living well with dementia: a National Dementia Strategy. London: Department of Health; 2009.
43. Department of Health. Prime Minister's Challenge on Dementia. Delivering major improvements in dementia care and research by 2015. London: Department of Health; 2012.
44. Department of Health. Prime Minister's Challenge on Dementia 2020. London: Department of Health; 2015.
45. Department of Health. G8 dementia summit declaration. London: Department of Health; 2013. https://www.gov.uk/government/publications/g8-dementia-summit-agreements/g8-dementia-summit-declaration

Chapter 2
Dementia: The Conduct of Anaesthesia

Stephen Alcorn and Gemma Alcorn

Introduction

While surgery and anaesthesia have been known to induce variable impairments in cognitive function for decades [1], the contribution of drugs delivered during anaesthesia has been relatively under-studied. The reasons underlying this dearth of research are myriad, however our incomplete understanding of dementia pathophysiology has undoubtedly hindered the study of these drugs' effects in this particular arena. Ethical and practical difficulties surrounding research on human cerebral tissue has necessitated a reliance on animal studies and human cell culture research which are useful, but ultimately imperfect models of human physiology and pharmacodynamics, particularly in the context of a disease spectrum affecting the function of an organ as complex and as relatively poorly understood as the human brain. Furthermore, a fully coherent understanding and classification of disorders of cognitive function in the postoperative period has not been developed; the relationship between

S. Alcorn (✉) · G. Alcorn
Western General Hospital, Edinburgh, UK
e-mail: stephen.alcorn@nhs.net

© Springer International Publishing AG, part of Springer Nature 2018
A. Severn (ed.), *Cognitive Changes after Surgery in Clinical Practice*, In Clinical Practice,
https://doi.org/10.1007/978-3-319-75723-0_2

emergence delirium, postoperative delirium (POD), postoperative cognitive dysfunction (POCD) and new onset dementia or neurocognitive disorder therefore remains unclear.

This chapter will attempt to outline an evidence-based assessment of the risks and benefits of those drugs and techniques available to anaesthetists who may be asked to deliver safe perioperative care to patients with potentially frail brains. Cardiac surgery, where the unique contributions of specific cardiac surgery-associated risk factors to POCD has been well-documented elsewhere [2], will not be specifically covered however many of the drugs discussed remain of relevance. Starting with pre-operative medications, and progressing chronologically through the patient's journey the chapter will conclude with management of pain and nausea.

Pre-operative Assessment

The pre-operative clinic or visit provides the anaesthetist with the opportunity to review patients' cognitive status and review their usual medications. Of particular interest in the context of cognitive impairment are drugs used in the treatment of dementia such as rivastigmine, donepezil and galantamine. These drugs are anticholinesterases and as such may interact with both neuromuscular blocking agents (NMBAs) and anticholinesterases used to reverse blockade [3–6]. Guidance on whether to continue or withhold these drugs in advance of scheduled anaesthesia is inconsistent, however a large retrospective study comparing patients taking these drugs with matched controls for whom they were not prescribed found no difference in outcome after hip fracture surgery [7]. On the other hand, abrupt cessation of these medicines can cause severe adverse cognitive and non-cognitive problems (e.g. paralytic ileus) [8, 9]. A pragmatic approach based on the existing evidence therefore would be to continue them throughout the perioperative period but prepare for potential interactions.

Polypharmacy in older adults is a major cause of morbidity [10] and where possible the anaesthetist may wish to consult specialist elderly medicine physicians or experienced pharmacists regarding other potential drug interactions in the perioperative period. The Beers criteria [11], a list of potentially inappropriate medications in older adults produced by the American Geriatrics Society is an invaluable resource. Many drugs are included in the list as a direct consequence of their anticholinergic activity; since dementia pathophysiology and central cholinergic transmission are inextricably linked [12] drugs with significant anticholinergic effect should be avoided where this is practical. Several anticholinergic burden scales are available (including, for example, the Magellan scale) which may assist with identifying drugs with obvious or more subtle anticholinergic side effects [13].

Patients with dementia are at increased risk of both cognitive and non-cognitive adverse postoperative outcomes [14]; this may include increased rates of falls, infection, discharge to long-term care facilities, and mortality. The elderly and cognitively impaired are also frequently affected by comorbid conditions and for these reasons it is important to consider the individual patient holistically when selecting pharmacological agents as part of an anaesthetic plan, since the effects of these drugs and their interactions with patients' comorbidities may only be detectable in the days or even weeks following the operative intervention.

Premedication

The use of routine benzodiazepine premedication is discouraged due to the increased potential for postoperative delirium, cognitive impairment, and falls [11, 12, 15, 16]. However, this advice can be tempered with clinical judgement since cognitively impaired patients (particularly those with more significant impairment) may suffer distress, anxiety and agitation in the unfamiliar environment of the anaesthetic room [17]. This distress may itself contribute to

POD. In the few cases where this is likely to be of benefit, for example where a confused elderly patient requires sedation for a regional anaesthetic technique, this should be limited to the lowest possible dose of a short acting agent such as propofol, alfentanil, or if necessary midazolam, titrated to effect.

The practice of premedication with anticholinergic agents is now fortunately rare: the effects of tertiary amines hyoscine, and indeed atropine, are mediated via central, as well as peripheral, cholinergic inhibition and thus they are highly likely to contribute to a worsening cognitive status. Drugs with quaternary amine structures such as glycopyrronium do not directly affect the central nervous system and are therefore the antimuscarinic of choice for premedication where, for example, reduction in airway secretions will be of benefit [18].

Regional Anaesthesia

The evidence to support improved outcomes with regional anaesthesia in populations at risk of cognitive impairment when compared to general anaesthesia is generally weak [16, 19, 20] however there are numerous confounding variables which may have prevented clear evidence of benefit or harm from being detected. Any positive effect which may be gained due to improved postoperative mobility or reduced postoperative opioid consumption may be offset by the use of benzodiazepines to facilitate block placement, or the development and subsequent insufficient treatment of hypotension following neuraxial block, leading to a number of adverse neurological and cardiovascular outcomes. Furthermore, not all studies of regional anaesthesia in this population have controlled for depth of sedation used, resulting in a lack of clear distinction between cohorts receiving general anaesthesia and those receiving both regional anaesthesia and deep sedation - which may be tantamount to general anaesthesia and has been shown to increase risk of POD [21].

One well-designed randomised study comparing the clinical progression of amnestic mild cognitive impairment (aMCI) and cerebrospinal fluid (CSF) markers associated with Alzheimer's disease found similar rates of both progression and disease markers in groups undergoing anaesthesia with either total intravenous anaesthesia (TIVA) or epidural anaesthesia for spinal surgery [22]. Both groups were comparable to nonsurgical control patients who were tested at the same time points, while those who underwent general anaesthesia with a volatile agent exhibited significantly increased levels of progression in their cognitive impairment at 2 years (although not to Alzheimer's disease), and increased CSF markers associated with the development of dementia relative to the other groups postoperatively. Regional anaesthesia might therefore be equivalent to TIVA and superior to volatile anaesthesia in appropriately selected members of the population at risk of postoperative cognitive impairment. Unfortunately the relative impracticality of performing regional anaesthesia in patients with significant pre-existing cognitive impairment without the use of sedative drugs be a serious handicap to its widespread application in patients with established dementia.

Induction of Anaesthesia

Propofol and thiopentone are both considered safe induction agents in populations at risk of dementia since neither drug has significant activity at central acetylcholine (ACh) receptors [16, 23] nor do they interfere with amyloid precursor protein (APP) metabolism in animal models [24]. Some controversy exists regarding dose modification of propofol in patients with pre-existing cognitive impairment as patients with lower mini-mental state examination (MMSE) scores have been found to require lower induction doses [25] however this is difficult to predict reliably. The literature therefore broadly recommends that usual dose modifications for elderly patients (e.g. up to 50% dose reduction as a slow bolus in the frail elderly) are used in this context [16].

Alternative induction agents such as etomidate and ketamine have been less thoroughly investigated with regard to their effect on postoperative cognitive function. Ketamine in particular remains controversial. It is of interest that it has been credited with reduction in POD after cardiac surgery [26] but this effect has not been consistently described [27]. Its clinical profile and propensity for hallucinations and nightmares is well known and several authors recommend avoiding this drug entirely due to increased POD risk [28, 29]. However this evidence remains based upon 'expert opinion' rather than any trial data. Large-scale trials evaluating the relationship between ketamine and cognitive dysfunction after surgery, outwith the context of cardiopulmonary bypass, are awaited. As both propofol and thiopentone are considered safe induction agents it may be wise to restrict alternative drugs to those situations where a clear benefit outweighs the potential risk.

NMBAs, both depolarizing and non depolarising such as suxamethonium, atracurium, rocuronium and vecuronium, all operate via their affinity for nicotinic acetylcholine receptors and hence their activity can be affected by the anticholinesterases used to treat dementia. Suxamethonium and mivacurium metabolism by pseudocholinesterase enzymes may also be affected, resulting in prolonged block in the presence of these drugs [4]. The phenomenon of Phase 2 depolarising block, long considered an obsolete, rarely observed and little known side effect of prolonged block after repeated or excessive suxamethonium administration, has become a practical issue both with depolarising agents and, if neostigmine is administered, after non-depolarising NMBAs even in the absence of suxamethonium in patients taking anticholinesterases for dementia [5]. Conversely and predictably, if no neostigmine is present, these anticholinesterases will confer resistance to non-depolarising agents [6].

In patients taking anticholinesterase medication, therefore, suxamethonium should be administered at the usual dose, while an increased dose of non-depolarising NMBAs should be considered, especially if rapid sequence intubation with rocuronium is planned [16]. In all cases where NMBAs are used for patients also taking anticholinesterases, neuromuscular stimulator monitoring is mandatory in order to quantify the potentially unpredictable response [20]. Sugammadex, a modified gamma-cyclodextrin, is a novel agent used for the reversal of aminosteroid (rocuronium or vecuronium) paralysis. It is specific for these NMBAs as its 3D structure (a tubular molecule with a hydrophobic internal cavity) traps these molecules via hydrophobic interactions, removing them from their site of action (i.e. the neuromuscular junction) and rapidly reverses their effect in a dose-dependent manner. The use of sugammadex to reverse neuromuscular blockade may be ideally suited to this population as it obviates the need for neostigmine and therefore any potential interaction. Similarly, the combination of rocuronium and potential reversal with sugammadex may be the safest strategy should rapid sequence induction be necessary in patients on dementia treatment as it additionally removes the risk of interaction with suxamethonium [20].

Maintenance of Anaesthesia

The question of whether volatile anaesthetic agents contribute to the development of POCD or POD, and if so, which agents are most or least culpable, is one of the most contentious in this field. When directly compared with total intravenous anaesthesia (TIVA), however, volatile agents have been consistently associated with worse cognitive outcomes. This includes increased POCD incidence [30], increased severity of POD [31], and progression of mild amnestic cognitive impairment [22]. No such complications have been attributed to the use of the anaesthetic gas nitrous oxide, used in conjunction with volatile agents [32] despite its possible effects on the central cholinergic system.

There is a reasonable body of evidence comparing individual volatile agents in order to ascertain which might be most useful, or least harmful, in this population. However, many of the studies yield contradictory results, often based on different cellular biomarkers whose clinical significance is not definitively established. Desflurane has been recommended by several authors over the older, more water soluble agents such as isoflurane and sevoflurane. In a number of clinical studies this has been associated with better outcomes in this population such as faster initial recovery, earlier mobilisation, and increased patient satisfaction [28, 33]. Increases in the brain biomarker $A\beta40$ in human cerebrospinal fluid have been seen with exposure to isoflurane which were not replicated with desflurane [34], while in the laboratory, deleterious effects such as caspase activation and generation of reactive oxygen species have been observed in animal neurons following isoflurane exposure which were not detected with desflurane [35]. It may therefore be reasonable to select desflurane where a volatile agent is indicated.

TIVA outcomes appear to be better than those seen with volatile agents. This may be the consequence of both avoidance of the deleterious neuronal changes which have been observed with volatiles, and the anti-inflammatory effect of propofol counteracting the surgical insult. There is some clinical evidence which may support this latter theory: decreased interleukin 6 (IL6), cortisol and catecholamine levels have been measured in patients undergoing TIVA anaesthesia when compared to control patients undergoing volatile-based anaesthesia [39, 40] although these particular studies failed to demonstrate improved cognitive outcomes associated with these changes.

Dosing of all anaesthetic agents - whether depth of anaesthesia is estimated with minimum alveolar concentration (MAC) values or measured with electroencephalographic data such as bispectral index (BIS) - may also affect cognitive outcomes. While it is currently unclear if or how exactly the anaesthetic requirements change in the cognitively impaired beyond that expected in those of increased age [25, 41] it is

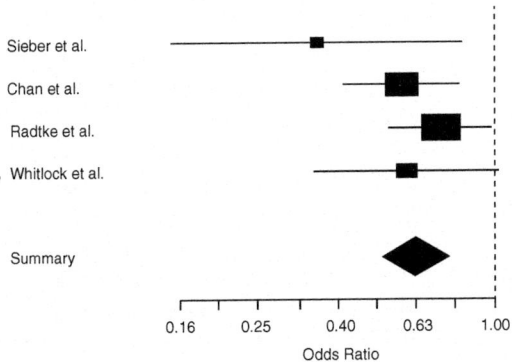

FIGURE 2.1 Meta-analysis of randomized controlled trials assessing postoperative delirium with intraoperative Bispectral Index (BIS) guidance of anesthesia compared with an alternative approach (i.e., usual care or an alternative protocol). Odds ratios <1 favor BIS guidance [21, 36–38]. (Reproduced with permission from Whitlock et al. 2014 [36])

apparent that deeper anaesthesia and higher doses of anaesthesia drugs increase the likelihood of POD and POCD, and that this problem can be diminished if anaesthesia depth is appropriately targeted using BIS monitoring [21, 36–38, 42–44].

This has been demonstrated in multiple controlled trials, however a meta-analysis illustrating the benefit of BIS use resulting in reduced POD incidence is perhaps one of the strongest indicators of its usefulness. In Fig. 2.1, a Forest plot depicts the results of several trials of BIS monitoring in a range of surgical contexts and clearly demonstrates the reduction in POD incidence.

Analgesia and Antiemetics

The effective management of pain appears to be a significant factor in the prevention of POD [45] and therefore appropriate multimodal strategies to improve postoperative analgesia should be employed. Regional techniques are discussed above, and these should be considered where indicated. Opioid analgesia is likely to provide the mainstay of most surgical analgesia strategies and is by no means contraindicated in this population, however dosing should be carefully considered and regularly reviewed. A 'start low and go slow' approach to opioid doses is routinely advocated; while this may reduce the risk of inadvertent overdosing, those who adopt this strategy must be particularly aware of the risk of underdosing leading to inadequately controlled pain and hence increased delirium risk. Pethidine and tramadol should be avoided as both are associated with POD [46, 47] but fentanyl, morphine and oxycodone are considered safe.

Adjunctive analgesic therapies such as clonidine and nonsteroidal anti-inflammatory drugs (NSAIDs) should be used with caution. Intravenous clonidine has effects on cognition which are generally positive, and it has shown promise in reducing delirium in intensive care, although this has not been shown in a meta-analysis evaluating its efficacy in preventing POD [48]. However, as a centrally-acting antihypertensive agent it may cause profound hypotension in combination with general anaesthesia and thereby adversely affect brain perfusion. Of note, it is strongly advised against as a first-line antihypertensive by the Beers criteria [11] due to the risk of symptomatic bradycardia and orthostatic hypotension. Where appropriate, however, a carefully titrated dose might reduce opioid requirements. NSAIDs are generally avoided in the elderly due to the substantial risks of gastrointestinal, renal, neurological and cardiovascular side effects. Although delirium and cognitive impairment are not specifically associated with NSAIDs, drowsiness, dizziness, and confusion have all been reported. If these drugs are to be used at all it should be for short courses only in selected patients. Paracetamol should be used to reduce opioid requirements and thereby opioid side-effects. Nefopam is associated with moderate anticholinergic activity and is therefore best avoided [13].

The use of dexmedetomidine, a highly specific α2-receptor agonist with analgesic, antisialagogue and sedative effects, in the intraoperative context is a relatively new development which may warrant further study. Its use in intensive care to treat and prevent delirium has been widely studied [49, 50] but evidence regarding its role in the operating theatre is currently limited. Several small studies which have been published have shown mixed results in preventing postoperative adverse cognitive outcomes, while a larger randomised trial has failed to demonstrate any benefit [51]. The hypothesis that by reducing doses of both volatile agents and opioids, and through anxiolytic and anti-inflammatory roles this drug might improve postoperative cognitive outcomes seems plausible, but this has not been proven and on the state of the current evidence it is not possible to recommend its administration in this context.

The incidence of postoperative nausea and vomiting (PONV) decreases with age such that many patients at risk of cognitive impairment will be significantly less likely to experience it than younger patient undergoing the same procedure [52]. Nevertheless, PONV risk should be assessed and appropriate prophylaxis administered if indicated. Several antiemetics carry significant anticholinergic burdens, including cyclizine, prochlorperazine and metoclopramide [11] which should be avoided. Ondansetron and low-dose dexamethasone are considered safe and are widely used in the elderly.

Conclusion

Although significant ground remains to be covered, an evidence-based approach to perioperative pharmacotherapy is much more firmly within our grasp than when adverse cognitive outcomes following anaesthesia were first described in the 1950s. Broadly speaking, central tenets of an ideal anaesthetic strategy would include avoidance of drugs known to be associated with delirium such as benzodiazepines, atropine and tramadol, use of short-acting agents and propofol-based anaesthesia where appropriate, and effective multimodal analgesia. These same principles would be applicable to the general management of a person known or suspected to have pre-existing cognitive dysfunction, from the point of view of preventing both the dangerous complication of delirium and potential aggravation of the long term cognitive deficit.

References

1. Bedford PD. Adverse cerebral effects of anaesthesia on old people. Lancet. 1955;2:259–63.
2. van Harten AE, Scheeren TWL, Absalom AR. A review of postoperative cognitive dysfunction and neuroinflammation associated with cardiac surgery and anaesthesia. Anaesthesia. 2012;67:280–93.
3. Crowe S, Collins L. Suxamethonium and donepezil : a cause of prolonged paralysis. Anesthesiology. 2003;98(2):574–5.
4. Bhardwaj A, Dharmavaram S, Wadhawan S, Sethi A, Bhadoria P. Donepezil: a cause of inadequate muscle relaxation and prolonged neuromuscular recovery. J Anaesthesiol Clin Pharmacol. 2011;27(2):247–8.
5. Sprung J, Castellani WJ, Srinivasan V, Udayashankar S. The effects of donepezil and neostigmine in a patient with unusual pseudocholinesterase activity. Anesth Analg. 1998;87(5):1203–5.
6. Pautola L, Reinikainen M. Donepezil/Rocuronium bromide interaction. Reactions Weekly. 2012;1423(1):21.
7. Seitz DP, Gill SS, Gruneir A, Austin PC, Anderson G, Reimer CL. Effects of cholinesterase inhibitors on postoperative outcomes of older adults with dementia undergoing hip fracture surgery. Am J Geriatr Psychiatry. 2011;19(9):803–13.
8. Bidzan L, Bidzan M. Withdrawal syndrome after donepezil cessation in a patient with dementia. Neurol Sci. 2012;33(6):1459–61.
9. Okazaki T, Furukawa K. Paralytic ileus after discontinuation of cholinesterase inhibitor. J Am Geriatr Soc. 2006;54(10):1620–1.
10. Sieber FE, Barnett SR. Preventing postoperative complications in the elderly. Anesthesiol Clin. 2011;29(1):83–97.
11. American Geriatrics Society Beers Criteria Update Expert Panel. American Geriatrics Society 2015 updated beers criteria for potentially inappropriate medication use in older adults. J

Am Geriatr Soc. 2015;63(11):2227–46. https://onlinelibrary.wiley.com/doi/epdf/10.1111/jgs.13702.

12. Kapoor M. Alzheimer's disease, anaesthesia and the cholinergic system. J Anesthesiol Clin Pharmacol. 2011;27(2):155–8.

13. Salahudeen MS, Duffull SB, Nishtala PS. Anticholinergic burden quantified by anticholinergic risk scales and adverse outcomes in older people: a systematic review. BMC Geriatr. 2015;15:31. https://doi.org/10.1186/s12877-015-0029-9.

14. Seitz DP, Gill SS, Gruneir A, Austin PC, Anderson GM, Bell CM, Rochon PA. Effects of dementia on postoperative outcomes of older adults with hip fractures: a population-based study. J Am Med Dir Assoc. 2014;15(5):334–41.

15. Arora SS, Gooch JL, Garcia PS. Postoperative cognitive dysfunction, Alzheimer's disease, and anaesthesia. Int J Neurosci. 2014;124(4):236–42.

16. Funder KS, Steinmetz J, Rasmussen LS. Anesthesia for the patient with dementia. J Alz Dis. 2010;22(S3):129–34.

17. Verborgh C. Anesthesia in patients with dementia. Curr Opin Anaesthesiol. 2004;17(3):277–83.

18. Burton DA, Nicholson G, Hall GM. Anaesthesia in patients with neurodegenerative conditions: special considerations. Drugs Aging. 2004;21(4):229–42.

19. Wu CL, Hsu W, Richman JM, Raja SN. Postoperative cognitive function as an outcome of regional anesthesia and analgesia. RAPM. 2004;29(3):257–68.

20. Funder KS, Steinmetz J, Rasmussen LS. Anaesthesia for the patient with dementia undergoing outpatient surgery. Curr Opin Anaesthesiol. 2009;22(6):712–7.

21. Sieber FE, Zakriya KJ, Gottschalk A, et al. Sedation depth during spinal anesthesia and the development of postoperative delirium in elderly patients undergoing hip fracture repair. Mayo Clin Proc. 2010;85(1):18–26.

22. Liu Y, Pan M, Ma Y, et al. Inhaled sevoflurane may promote progression of amnestic mild cognitive impairment: a prospective, randomized parallel-group study. Am J Med Sci. 2013;345(5):355–60.

23. Pratico C, Quattrone D, Lucent T, Amato A, Penna O, Roscitano C, Fodale V. Drugs of anesthesia acting on central cholinergic system may cause post-operative cognitive dysfunction and delirium. Med Hypoth. 2005;65(5):972–82.

24. Palotas M, Palotas A, Bjelik A, Pakaski M, Hugyecz M, Janka Z, Kalman J. Effect of general anesthetics on amyloid precursor

protein and mRNA levels in the rat brain. Neurochem Res. 2005;30(8):1021–6.

25. Erdogan MA, Demirbilek S, Erdil F, Aydogan MS, Ozturk E, Togal T, Ersoy MO. The effects of cognitive impairment on anaesthetic requirement in the elderly. Eur J Anesthesiol. 2012;29(7):326–31.

26. Hudetz JA, Patterson KM, Iqbal Z, Gandhi SD, Byrne AJ, Hudetz AG, Warltier DC, Pagel PS. Ketamine attenuates delirium after cardiac surgery with cardiopulmonary bypass. J Cardiothorac Vasc Anesth. 2009;23:651–7.

27. Bilotta F, Gelb AW, Stazi E, Titi L, Paoloni FP, Rosa G. Pharmacological perioperative neuroprotection: a qualitative review of randomized controlled trials. Br J Anaesth. 2013;110(S1):113–20.

28. Rudra A, Chatterjee S, Sengupta S. Alzheimer's disease and anaesthesia. J Anaesthesiol Clin Pharm. 2007;23(4):357–64.

29. Malinovsky JM, Hamidi A, Lelarge C, Boulay-Malinovsky C. Spécificités de la prise en charge anesthésique chez les patients souffrant de maladie neurologique : éclairage sur l'anesthésie locorégionale. Presse Med. 2014;43(7–8):756–64.

30. Cai Y, Hu H, Liu P, et al. Association between the apolipoprotein E4 and postoperative cognitive dysfunction in elderly patients undergoing intravenous anesthesia and inhalation anesthesia. Anesthesiology. 2012;116(1):84–93.

31. Tang N, Ou C, Liu Y, Zuo Y, Bai Y. Effect of inhalational anaesthetic on postoperative cognitive dysfunction following radical rectal resection in elderly patients with mild cognitive impairment. J Int Med Res. 2014;42(6):1252–61.

32. Leung JM, Sands LP, Vaurio LE, Wang Y. Nitrous oxide does not change the incidence of postoperative delirium or cognitive decline in elderly surgical patients. Br J Anaesth. 2006;96(6):754–60.

33. Rörtgen D, Kloos J, Fries M, et al. Comparison of early cognitive function and recovery after desflurane or sevoflurane anaesthesia in the elderly: a double-blind randomized controlled trial. Br J Anaesth. 2010;104(2):167–74.

34. Zhang B, Tian M, Zheng H, Zhen Y, Yue Y, Li T, Li S, Marcantonio ER, Xie Z. Effects of anesthetic isoflurane and desflurane on human cerebrospinal fluid Aβ and τ level. Anesthesiology. 2013;119(1):52–60.

35. Zhang Y, Xu Z, Wang H, Dong Y, Shi HN, Culley D, Crosby G, Marcantonio ER, Tanzi R. Anesthetics isoflurane and Desflurane

differently affect mitochondrial function, learning, and memory. Ann Neurol. 2012;71(5):687–98.

36. Whitlock EL, Torres BA, Lin N, Helsten DL, Nadelson MR, Mashour GA, Avidan MS. Postoperative delirium in a substudy of cardiothoracic surgical patients in the BAG-RECALL clinical trial. Anesth Analg. 2014;118(4):809–17.

37. Chan MTV, Cheng BCP, Lee TMC, Gin T. BIS-guided anesthesia decreases postoperative delirium and cognitive decline. J Neurosurg Anesth. 2013;25(1):33–42.

38. Radtke FM, Franck M, Lindner J, Krüger S, Wernecke KD, Spies CD. Monitoring depth of anaesthesia in a randomized trial decreases the rate of postoperative delirium but not postoperative cognitive dysfunction. Br J Anaesth. 2013;110(Suppl 1):i98–105.

39. Tang JX, Baranov D, Hammond M, Shaw LM, Eckenhoff MF, Eckenhoff RG. Human CSF Alzheimer and inflammatory biomarkers after anesthesia and surgery. Anesthesiology. 2011;115(4):727–32.

40. Deiner S, Lin HM, Bodansky D, Silverstein J, Sano M. Do stress markers and anesthetic technique predict delirium in the elderly? Dement Geriatr Cogn Disord. 2014;38(5–6):366–74.

41. Perez-Protto S, Geube M, Ontaneda D, Dalton JE, Kurz A, Sessler DI. Sensitivity to volatile anesthetics in patients with dementia: a case-control analysis. Can J Anesth. 2014;61(7):611–8.

42. Siddiqi N, Harrison JK, Clegg A, Teale EA, Young J, Taylor J, Simpkins SA. Interventions for preventing delirium in hospitalised patients. Cochrane Database Syst Rev. 2016;3:CD005563. https://doi.org/10.1002/14651858.CD005563.pub3.

43. Moyce Z, Rodseth RN, Biccard BM. The efficacy of perioperative interventions to decrease postoperative delirium in non-cardiac surgery: a systematic review and meta-analysis. Anaesthesia. 2014;69(3):259–69.

44. Ballard C, Jones E, Gauge N, Aarsland D, Nelson OB, Saxby BK, Lowery D, Corbett A, Wesnes K, Katsaiti E, Arden J, Amaoko D, Prophet N, Purushothaman B, Green D. Optimised Anaesthesia to reduce post operative cognitive decline (POCD) in older patients undergoing elective surgery, a randomised controlled trial. PLoS One. 2012;7(6):e37410.

45. Vaurio LE, Sands LP, Wang Y, Mullen EA, Leung JM. Postoperative delirium: the importance of pain and pain management. Anesth Analg. 2006;102(4):1267–73.

46. Marcantonio ER, Juarez G, Goldman L, Mangione CM, Ludwig LE, Lind L, Katz N, Cook EF, Orav EJ, Lee TH. The relationship of postoperative delirium with psychoactive medications. JAMA. 1994;272(19):1518–22.
47. Brouquet A, Cudennec T, Benoist S, Moulias S, Beauchet A, Penna C, Teillet L, Nordlinger B. Impaired mobility, ASA status and administration of tramadol are risk factors for postoperative delirium in patients aged 75 years or more after major abdominal surgery. Ann Surg. 2010;251(4):259–65.
48. Zhang H, Lu Y, Liu M, Zou Z, Wang L, Xu FY, Shi XY. Strategies for prevention of postoperative delirium: a systematic review and meta-analysis of randomized trials. Crit Care. 2013;17(2):R47. https://doi.org/10.1186/cc12566.
49. Jakob SM, Ruokonen E, Grounds RM, Sarapohja T, Garratt C, Pocock SJ, Bratty JR, Takala J. Dexmedetomidine for long-term sedation investigators FT. Dexmedetomidine vs midazolam or Propofol for sedation during prolonged mechanical ventilation: two randomized controlled trials. JAMA. 2012;307(11):1151–60.
50. Reade MC, O'Sullivan K, Bates S, Goldsmith D, Ainslie WR, Bellomo R. Dexmedetomidine vs. haloperidol in delirious, agitated, intubated patients: a randomised open-label trial. Crit Care. 2009;13(3):R75. https://doi.org/10.1186/cc7890.
51. Deiner S, Luo X, Lin HM, Sessler DI, Saager L, Sieber FE, Lee HB, Sano M. The Delirium Writing Group, Jankowski C, Bergese SD, Candiotti K, Flaherty JH, Arora H, Shander A, Rock P. Intraoperative infusion of dexmedetomidine for prevention of postoperative delirium and cognitive dysfunction in elderly patients undergoing major elective noncardiac surgery: a randomised clinical trial. JAMA Surg. 2017;152(8):e171505.
52. Apfel CC, Heidrich FM, Jukar-Rao S, Jalota L, Hornuss C, Whelan RP, Zhang K, Cakmakkaya OS. Evidence-based analysis of risk factors for postoperative nausea and vomiting. Br J Anaesth. 2012;109(5):742–53.

Chapter 3
Epidemiology, Mechanisms and Consequences of Postoperative Cognitive Dysfunction

Daniele Bryden

Introduction

Cognitive decline in the perioperative period can be easily dismissed as not a direct anaesthetic issue, partly because it is difficult to confirm clear linkages between a chosen anaesthetic technique and any cognitive decline and partly because agreed definitions of the spectrum of conditions that are understood as cognitive decline are lacking. However despite this, every anaesthetist will recognise the patient on their post op visit who is not mentally quite the same person they visited prior to surgery: often elderly, having undergone a significant surgical procedure, perhaps as an emergency and with ongoing issues from their pre exisiting co-morbidities

D. Bryden
Critical Care Department, Sheffield Teaching Hospitals NHS FT, Sheffield, UK
e-mail: daniele.bryden@sth.nhs.uk

© Springer International Publishing AG, part of Springer Nature 2018
A. Severn (ed.), *Cognitive Changes after Surgery in Clinical Practice*, In Clinical Practice, https://doi.org/10.1007/978-3-319-75723-0_3

eg polypharmacy, sepsis, anaemia. What part can the anaesthetic have had in what was probably an inevitable decline, and which may turn out to have no long term consequences anyway?

This chapter will provide an introduction to the spectrum of disorders that are understood as post operative cognitive dysfunction (POCD) and will illustrate why anaesthetists should consider post operative cognitive dysfunction as a significant risk for many patients and should plan their anaesthetic management and patient counselling accordingly.

What Is Post Operative Cognitive Dysfunction?

A patient with POCD has a significant detectable decline from baseline level of performance on at least one neuropsychological domain: POCD as an entity is a disorder of thinking and cognition after surgery. Whilst the tests for detecting POCD are validated, the definition of the condition is not, neither the International Classification of Disease (ICD-10) or the Diagnostic and Statistical Manual of Mental Disorders (DSM-V) list the condition as a distinct entity. A consensus definition is needed and is currently being refined, so in the interim it may be easiest thought of as a neurocognitive disorder with an as yet unspecified aetiology that begins 7 days to 1 year after surgery [1].

The earliest form of cognitive dysfunction observed in the postoperative period is delirium. Delirium is an acute confusional state with disturbed thinking and environmental inattention and is considered to occur between 24 and 96 h after surgery. Delirium is discussed elsewhere in this book but has not yet been definitively linked to long term cognitive impairment [2] and it is not necessary to have had delirium before developing POCD.

Whereas early POCD may be observed in up to 10% of elderly patients for up to 3 months postoperatively, symptoms that persist for 6–12 months are considered indicative of a more persistent POCD or long term cognitive impairment. Many of the studies examining longer term POCD lack longitudinal follow up, matched controls or take account of the learning effects of neurocognitive testing [3]. Running in parallel to the development of any new cases of POCD are patients who may have undiagnosed dementia or other chronic decline in cognitive function.

Dementia is expected to double in incidence in the next 30 years in the UK [4]. Forty-eight percent of unplanned hospital admissions in those over 80 years of age have dementia and common reasons for admission include hip fracture, chronic limb ischaemia and stroke. Dementia and its impact for anaesthetic management is also discussed as a separate chapter in this book.

For many people however, any persistent degree of cognitive impairment would be concerning, but some authors have suggested that in older patients receiving general anaesthesia, there are increased risks of developing dementia. Currently the evidence base is not clear, which makes counselling patients as to their individual risk of developing POCD potentially problematic [5]. There is variation in the tests used to assess POCD and in their timing and interpretation. In addition the point at which testing is performed may give only a short observation of an individual's cognitive trajectory but will not differentiate between someone whose cognitive trajectory is worsened, unchanged or even improved by a surgical procedure. Figure 3.1 illustrates how cognitive trajectory measured at only 2 points in the perioperative period may not give a true picture.

Despite the problems of timing of testing, the Z score is emerging as the best way of analysing changes in cognitive function in the perioperative period. The Z score takes into account the pre and post operative cognitive decline of an individual and compares it to a control population: it is considered abnormal if the Z score is two standard deviations from the mean [6].

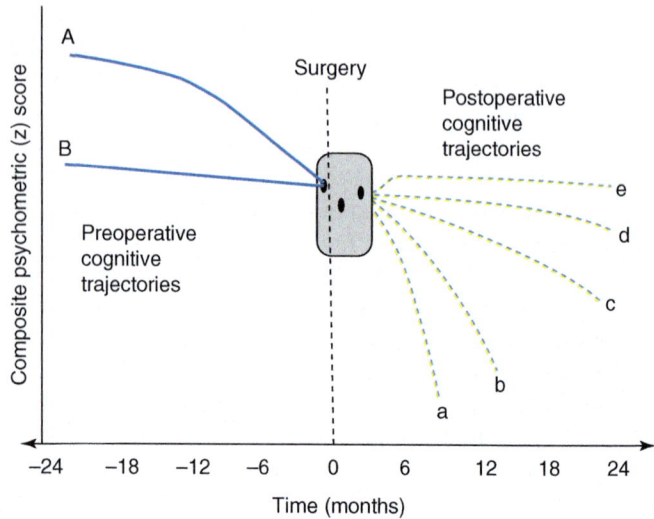

FIGURE 3.1 Preoperative and postoperative cognitive trajectories. This illustrates possible preoperative and postoperative cognitive trajectories for a single patient. Curve (A) illustrates a patient experiencing cognitive decline prior to surgery whilst in contrast curve (B) represents a patient with relatively stable cognitive function. A number of postoperative trajectory curves (a-e are possible). In patient (A), curve (b) represents a continuation of the preoperative trend. Curve (a) would be an acceleration of cognitive decline and curve (c) would be a reduction in cognitive decline, or even cognitive improvement. Without knowing Patient A's cognitive trajectory in the pre-op period, curves (a–c) could all be interpreted as POCD. For patient (B), curve (c) shows POCD, curve (d) is no change from the preoperative course, and curve (e) represents a cognitive improvement. Of note curve c can be interpreted as relative cognitive *improvement* for patient (A) and relative cognitive *decline* for patient (B), hence the importance of knowing the preoperative cognitive trajectory for an individual. (Reproduced with permission from Avidan and Nadelson [5])

Currently there is no clarity as to whether POCD is part of a continuum that leads to the development of dementia or a separate disease process and there is a need to resolve these relationships.

Epidemiology of POCD

The literature quotes a wide range of prevalence of POCD in part due to population heterogeneity as well as issues of definition and testing already highlighted. In patients undergoing hip surgery the prevalence has been quoted at 22% but in cardiac surgery has been reported as high as 60%: clearly a significant number of people may be affected at some point in the post op period [7]. Systematic review has indicated a prevalence of 12% in a general, adult, non cardiac surgical population [8] – the utility of such a figure for individual patient counselling is doubtful.

Identification of risk factors is also problematic but current evidence from published studies is summarised in Table 3.1.

It is not clear whether POCD is a reversible condition or is progressive, but there is no current evidence that would suggest it is irreversible. MacLullich reviewed studies published since 2004 of over 2000 hospitalised patients in total and suggested a link between early cognitive dysfunction and more long term impairment [9]. A more recent study reporting the follow up of a subgroup of participants in an international multicentre study on long term cognitive dysfunction

TABLE 3.1 Potential perioperative risk factors for POCD identified from published studies

Peri-operative risk factors for POCD	
Prior patient factors	**Perioperative factors**
Increasing age	Type of surgery: cardiac, orthopaedic or vascular
Low education level	Post operative respiratory complications, infections
History of cerebrovascular accident with no residual impairment	Time spent with Bispectral Index Measured <40 (inconclusive)
Prior Cognitive Impairment	
Poor functional status	

(ISPCOD 1) found no association between a diagnosis of POCD at 1 week or 3 months after surgery and more long term cognitive impairment or dementia [10].

Mechanisms of POCD

The mechanisms by which POCD occurs have been largely unstudied, with most research focusing on biological linkages between use of volatile anaesthetic agents and protein changes in the brain associated with dementia type conditions eg Alzheimer's disease and subsequent neuronal death. Moreover in older animals the volatile anaesthetic agents isoflurane and sevoflurane damage the brain vascular endothelium and increase blood brain barrier permeability allowing cytokines and pro-inflammatory mediators access to neuronal cells with resultant neuronal dysfunction. The translation between cell culture and animal study models to human biology is not yet made, but does at least provide some suggestion as to how administration of anaesthetic agents in an otherwise well controlled anaesthetic may produce POCD [11].

Diffusion weighted MRI scanning has provided an additional suggested mechanism of microemboli occurring from the surgical site or use of cardiopulmonary bypass circuits and causing cerebral infarctions. Several studies have demonstrated new lesions but linkage between the lesions, detectable test changes and POCD has not been made [12].

The evidence for intra-operative potentially modifiable anaesthetic factors is also weak, with no association shown between global hypotension and hypoxia and POCD in a major international study on post operative cognitive dysfunction [13] but some suggestion in cardiac surgical populations that cerebral hypoperfusion or hypoxia may be contributory [14]. Older people with evidence of brain pathology eg dementia are more sensitive to the hypnotic effects of anaesthesia and it is generally recommended that intraoperative monitoring of depth of anaesthesia and cardiovascular physiology is adopted. There is weak evidence that processed EEG monitoring reduces the incidence of POCD along with use of near infrared spectroscopy to avoid low cerebral oxygen saturations [15].

Consequences of POCD- Why Prevention Matters

Whilst POCD may lack definition and clarity of mechanism, there is evidence to suggest it is associated with increased mortality, impaired quality of life and loss of employment [16]. As such POCD should be managed pre-emptively within a package of measures designed to prevent its occurrence or minimise its impact. This should include a willingness to discuss risks with patients of a condition that whilst not clearly defined, has considerable concern for many individuals. Most UK centres have not yet adopted such an approach to proactively managing any form of POCD, but may do so with the publication in 2018 of guidance on perioperative care of dementia patients from the Association of Anaesthetists of Great Britain and Ireland.

Detection of cognitive impairment pre-operatively is a significant risk factor for postoperative decline and patients over the age of 65 years should be routinely screened if possible, to allow for decision making and modification of treatment plans [17] as well as referral for more formal cognitive testing. The Addenbrooke's Cognitive Exam (ACE-R) is one example of a validated test used by occupational health physicians that can be used to trigger a more detailed neuropsychiatric assessment or investigation. Currently funding, training and time constraints are barriers to more widespread adoption of this planning but development of Commissioning for Quality and Innovation (CQUIN) guidance on Dementia/Delirium by NHS England may also promote more awareness and widen adoption [18].

Additional assessment should include review of alcohol and smoking history with modification if necessary and clear planning for medication use or omission [19] (Fig. 3.2).

Meta analysis of involvement of care of the elderly physicians in comprehensive medication reviews has shown improved cognition after emergency admission to hospital so may be considered to be of benefit [20]. Current logic would suggest that packages of care designed for frail elderly patients would be beneficial and that particular attention should be paid to optimisation of general population vascular risk factors such as smoking, diabetes and hypertension as modifiable factors in reducing the incidence of POCD.

Correction of anaemia, electrolyte imbalances and reduction in fasting times for clear fluids are additional factors of general benefit in the at risk groups.

The randomized controlled PREHAB study currently being conducted in Canada is examining the impact of preoperative rehabilitation prior to cardiac surgery [21]. Cognitive function is being assessed as part of this trial and may provide some useful information as to whether a package of preoperative cardiovascular health measures can have a positive impact prior to undergoing cardiac surgery, a known high risk insult for POCD.

Trials of anaesthetic technique are heterogenous and comparisons are difficult: there is no evidence to favour one volatile agent over another, neuraxial anaesthesia over general or ultra short acting opiates (remifentanil) over other short acting agents (fentanyl). There is a clear need for well designed trials in this area, and in the interim, the best anaesthetic advice is to manage the patient using the most suitable and stable technique for that patient in that anaesthetist's hands.

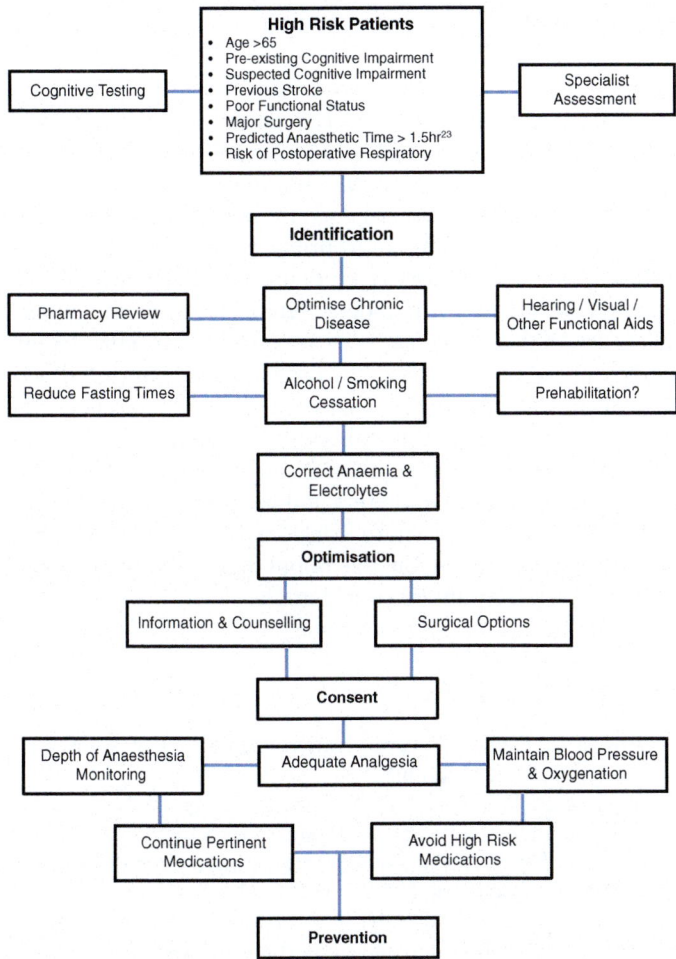

FIGURE 3.2 Suggested Flow Diagram for the Perioperative Process of Patients at High Risk of POCD. (Developed by C. Webb, M. Needham, D. Bryden). (Reproduced with permission from Needham MJ and Webb C [19])

Conclusions

Post operative cognitive dysfunction is a condition where increasing awareness and concern regarding individual patient risks now needs to be matched with agreed definitions and assessment tools and processes for diagnosis. Pre-operative assessment clinics could take up the challenge of widening screening and providing appropriate counselling in addition to linking in to packages of care that can be developed in conjunction with care of the elderly physicians and old age psychiatrists. Whilst there is no clear evidence to point to any single anaesthetic technique as protective or associated with long term damage, every anaesthetist should consider the impact of their planned technique for a patient on the likelihood of them developing POCD and make adjustments to drugs, physiological parameters and monitoring accordingly.

POCD is an area where considerably more research is needed as the impact on the population in individual and economic terms could be considerable.

References

1. Brown C, Deiner S. Perioperative cognitive protection. Br J Anaesth. 2016;117(S3):iii52–61.
2. Williamson WK, Nicoloff A. Functional outcome after open repair of abdominal aortic aneurysm. J Vasc Surg. 2001;33:913–20.
3. Tsai TL, Sands L. An update on postoperative cognitive dysfunction. Adv Anesth. 2010;28(1):269–84.
4. Department of Health. (2013). Dementia A state of the nation report on dementia care and support in England.
5. Nadelson MR, Sanders R. Perioperative cognitive trajectory in adults. Br J Anaesth. 2014;112(3):440–51.
6. Rudolph JL, Schreiber K. Measurement of post-operative cognitive dysfunction after cardiac surgery: a systematic review. Acta Anaesthesiol Scand. 2010;54(6):663–77.
7. Chow WB, Rosenthal R. Optimal preoperative assessment of the geriatric surgical patient: a best practices guideline from the American College of Surgeons national surgical quality

improvement program and the American Geriatrics Society. J Am Coll Surg. 2012;215(4):453–66.

8. Paredes S, Cortínez L. Post-operative cognitive dysfunction at 3 months in adults after non-cardiac surgery: a qualitative systematic review. Acta Anaesthesiologica Scandinavica. 2016;60:1043–58.

9. MacLullich AMJ, Beaglehole A. Delirium and long-term cognitive impairment. Int Rev Psychiatry. 2009;21(1):30–42.

10. Steinmetz J, Siersma V. Is postoperative cognitive dysfunction a risk factor for dementia? A cohort follow-up study. Br J Anaesth. 2013;110(S1):i92–7.

11. Fodale V, Santamaria L. Anaesthetics and postoperative cognitive dysfunction: a pathological mechanism mimicking Alzheimer's disease. Anaesthesia. 2010;65(4):388–95.

12. Sun X, Lindsay J. Silent brain injury after cardiac surgery: a review: cognitive dysfunction and magnetic resonance imaging diffusion-weighted imaging findings. J Am Coll Cardiol. 2012;60(9):791–7.

13. Moller JT, Cluitmans P. Long-term postoperative cognitive dysfunction in the elderly: ISPOCD1 study. Lancet. 1998;351:857–61.

14. van Harten AE, Scheeren T. A review of postoperative cognitive dysfunction and neuroinflammation associated with cardiac surgery and anaesthesia. Anaesthesia. 2012;67(3):280–93.

15. Ballard C, Jones E. Optimised anaesthesia to reduce post operative cognitive decline (POCD) in older patients undergoing elective surgery, a randomised controlled trial. PLoS One. 2012;7:e37410.

16. Berger M, Nadler J. Postoperative cognitive dysfunction: minding the gaps in our knowledge of a common postoperative complication in the elderly. Anesthesiol Clin. 2015;33:517–50.

17. Evered L, Scott D. Cognitive decline associated with anesthesia and surgery in the elderly: does this contribute to dementia prevalence? Curr Opin Psychiatry. 2017;30:220–6.

18. NHS England/Contracting and Incentives Team. 2015. Commissioning for quality and innovation guidance 2015/2016. Retrieved January 28, 2018, from https://www.england.nhs.uk/wp-content/uploads/2015/03/9-cquin-guid-2015-16.pdf.

19. Needham MJ, Webb C. Postoperative cognitive dysfunction and dementia: what weneed to know and do. British Journal of Anaesthesia. 2017;119(Suppl 1):115–25.

20. Ellis G, Whitehead M. Comprehensive geriatric assessment for older adults admitted to hospital: meta-analysis of randomised controlled trials. BMJ. 2011;343:d6553.
21. Stammers AN, Kehler D. Protocol for the PREHAB study-Pre-operative Rehabilitation for reduction of Hospitalization After coronary Bypass and valvular surgery: a randomised controlled trial. BMJ Open. 2015;5(3):e007250.

Chapter 4
Assessment of Cognitive Function

Andrew Larner

Introduction: The Need for Effective Cognitive Assessment

The prevalence and incidence of cognitive decline is predicted to increase dramatically with the ageing of the world population, since increasing age is a significant unmodifiable risk factor for cognitive disorders. The assessment of cognitive complaints and the identification of preclinical cognitive impairment which might progress to dementia are therefore likely to become clinical skills of increasing importance and relevance in future years, the more so if effective symptomatic, disease modifying and preventative therapies for cognitive impairment and dementia disorders are defined. Guides to cognitive assessment which are accessible to, and designed for use by, all clinicians are available [1]. This chapter aims to give a brief overview of the important cognitive domains and their assessment, with a particular focus on the use of cognitive screening instruments, the deployment of which may be

A. Larner
Cognitive Function Clinic, Walton Centre for Neurology
and Neurosurgery, Liverpool, UK
e-mail: a.larner@thewaltoncentre.nhs.uk

© Springer International Publishing AG, part of Springer
Nature 2018
A. Severn (ed.), *Cognitive Changes after Surgery in Clinical Practice*, In Clinical Practice,
https://doi.org/10.1007/978-3-319-75723-0_4

required if policies to screen for cognitive impairment become widely adopted.

Assessment of the Domains of Cognitive Function

Cognitive testing may broadly be divided into "bedside testing" administered by a clinician, and "formal" neuropsychological assessment administered by a trained clinical neuropsychologist. Although there is some overlap in terms of purpose, it may generally be said that the former is relatively brief and aims to answer a clinical question, whereas the latter is more exhaustive and probes to a finer degree performance in the various aspects or "domains" of cognitive function (the "instruments of the mind"). "Bedside" cognitive testing may answer the clinical requirements in many patients with cognitive complaints, with formal neuropsychological assessment being reserved for more complex and/or challenging cases. Formal neuropsychological assessment is required to quantify accurately performance on various tests, to allow comparison with age-matched controls, and to assess change over time when repeated after a suitable time interval (usually ≥6 months) [2–4]. Since availability of formal neuropsychological assessment as a clinical resource is limited, the focus here will be on so-called "bedside" testing (although this is best undertaken in a quiet environment, away from the bedside, free of distractions which might adversely impact patient test performance).

The cognitive domains amenable to examination by cognitive assessment are typically labelled as:

- Global intelligence (IQ)
- Memory
- Language
- Perception (visual, auditory, tactile)
- Praxis (skilled learned motor movements)
- Executive functions (sometimes labelled "frontal lobe functions")

These domains may be considered as nodes within an extended network which are specialised for particular functions, all of which work in concert, rather than isolation, to produce what we understand as consciousness [5].

Meaningful assessment of these cognitive domains cannot be undertaken if attentional mechanisms are impaired. Attention, or concentration, is a non-uniform, distributed cognitive function which may be defined as that component of consciousness which allots awareness or vigilance to particular sensory stimuli, allowing them to reach awareness or salience. Attentional resources are finite and hence may be directed to or focussed on some sensory channels but not others, implying that attention is effortful, selective, and closely linked to intention. Impairment of attentional mechanisms is the hallmark of delirium, which may or may not be associated with evident impairments of level of consciousness.

Bedside tests which can probe different brain regions, and hence permit some degree of localization and lateralization of impaired cognitive function, include:

- Verbal and semantic (object meaning) memory – L temporal lobe
- Visual memory and face recognition – R temporal lobe
- Naming and reading – L hemisphere
- Praxis, calculation, spelling, digit span – L parietal lobe
- Interpretation of fragmented objects and letters, dot counting – R parietal lobe
- Cognitive estimates, verbal fluency – frontal lobes

Many of these focalized tests are incorporated into the various commonly used cognitive screening instruments (see next section). Whilst these generic instruments are commonly used to provide a total cognitive "score", specific diagnosis is often dependent upon characterising not only the extent but also the focality of any deficits, which may have positive predictive value for different diseases (e.g. recall memory typically affected early and disproportionately in Alzheimer's disease; visuospatial functions in dementia with Lewy bodies;

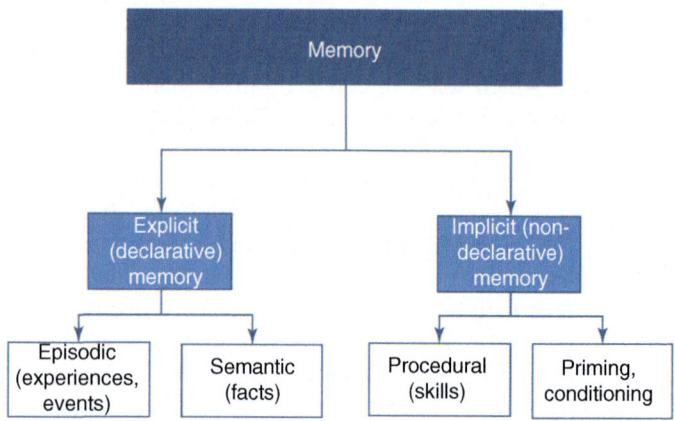

FIGURE 4.1 A simplified taxonomy of memory processes

linguistic and executive functions in the various forms of frontotemporal lobar degeneration).

The definition of cognitive domains permits a structured approach to the clinical assessment of cognitive function. Tests devoted to the assessment of each of the individual domains are available, but as the most common cognitive complaint encountered by clinicians relates to poor memory, the focus here will be on memory testing.

Memory is a non-uniform, distributed cognitive function within which a number of functional subdivisions may be differentiated. Current taxonomies of memory make a distinction between declarative memories (also known as explicit or conscious memory) and non-declarative memories (also known as implicit, procedural, unconscious, memory). "Working memory" or immediate memory is better conceptualized as an aspect of attentional mechanisms (Fig. 4.1).

Memory complaints usually relate to autobiographical or episodic declarative memories, and hence these are the usual focus of memory assessments. These are most commonly undertaken in "bedside testing" in the context of the administration of cognitive screening instruments.

Cognitive Screening Instruments, with a Focus on Memory Testing

As the name implies, cognitive screening instruments are designed for cognitive screening assessment. Hence they are not diagnostic tests, merely indicators of which patients with cognitive symptoms may be reassured and which may require further investigations. Many cognitive screening instruments are available [6–8], and most can be administered within a few minutes, usually no more than 20–30, sometimes less than 5 min (Box 4.1).

What features are desirable in cognitive screening instruments for effective cognitive assessment? Criteria for such instruments were specified by the Research Committee of the American Neuropsychiatric Association (Table 4.1) [9, 10].

Memory testing may examine either anterograde memory (new information given at the time of testing) or retrograde memory (information previously committed to memory, such

---

Box 4.1 Approximate times to administer some of the most commonly used cognitive screening instruments

Clock Drawing Test: <1 min
Six-item Cognitive Impairment Test (6CIT): 2–3 min
Abbreviated Mental Test Score (AMTS): <5 min
Mini-Mental State Examination (MMSE): 5–10 min
Mini-Addenbrooke's Cognitive Examination (MACE):
5–10 min
Test Your Memory (TYM) test
(self-administered under medical supervision):
5–10 min
DemTect: 8–10 min
Montreal Cognitive Assessment (MoCA): 10–15 min
Addenbrooke's Cognitive Examination (ACE-III):
15–20 min

TABLE 4.1 Desirable features for cognitive screening instruments

1. Should take <15 min to administer by a clinician at any level of training.

2. Should sample all major cognitive domains, including memory, attention/concentration, executive function, visual-spatial skills, language, and orientation (see Box 4.2 for the item content of some of the most commonly used cognitive screening instruments).

3. Should be reliable, with adequate test-retest and inter-rater validity.

4. Should be able to detect cognitive disorders (i.e. are sufficiently sensitive) which are commonly encountered by neuropsychiatrists (this latter point a reflection of the constituency drawing up the criteria).

5. Ease of test administration: not much equipment should be required for administration beyond a pencil and paper, or laptop computer (touch screen).

6. Ease of test interpretation: clear test cut-offs should be specified, such that particular test scores should lead to particular actions (i.e. the test is operationalised), such as patient reassurance, continued monitoring of cognitive function over specified time periods, or immediate initiation of further investigations and/or treatment. This recommendation stems in part from the fact that scores on cognitive screening instruments are non-linear (they have no specific units), some test items are more informative/better predictors than others, and test scores are subject to ceiling and floor effects.

7. Possibility for repeated (longitudinal) use of the test. The availability of variant forms of cognitive screening instruments may permit repeated testing over time whilst avoiding the potential pitfalls of practice effects [11]. Interpretation of repeat testing may be facilitated by provision of reliable change indices (RCI) from normative population studies [12].

Box 4.2 Item content of some of the most commonly used cognitive screening instruments: MMSE, MoCA, ACE-III, MACE

	MMSE	MoCA	ACE-III	MACE
Orientation: Time	5	4	5	4
Orientation: Place	5	2	5	–
Registration	3	–	3	–
Attention/ Concentration (serial 7 s, DLROW)	5	6 (3 for serial 7 s; 2 repeating digits forwards or backwards; 1 tapping to letter A)	5 (serial 7 s only)	–
Memory: Recall	3	5	3	–
Memory: Anterograde memory (name and address)	–	–	19	14
Memory: Retrograde memory	–	–	4	–
Verbal fluency: Letters and Animals in 1 min	–	1 (letter)	14	7 (letter or animals in different versions)
Language: Naming	2	3	12	–
Language: Comprehension	4	–	7	–
Language: Repetition	1	2	4	–

(continued)

Box 4.2 (continued)

	MMSE	MoCA	ACE-III	MACE
Language: Reading	–	–	1	–
Language: Writing	1	–	2	–
Visuospatial abilities: Intersecting pentagons	1	–	1 (intersecting lemnisci)	–
Visuospatial abilities: Wire (Necker) cube	–	1	2	–
Visuospatial abilities: Clock drawing	–	3	5	5
Visuospatial abilities: Trail making	–	1	–	–
Perceptual abilities: Dot counting	–	–	4	–
Perceptual abilities: Fragmented letters	–	–	4	–
Abstraction	–	2	–	–
Total Score	**30**	**30**	**100**	**30**

as past life events or facts). In anterograde memory testing the initial presentation is called the registration phase, and consists of material such as:

- a series of unrelated words, as in the Mini-Mental State Examination (MMSE) [13], the Montreal Cognitive Assessment (MoCA) [14], and DemTect [15];

- a fictional name and address, as in the Abbreviated Mental Test Score (AMTS) [16], the Six-item Cognitive Impairment Test (6CIT) [17], and the various iterations of the Addenbrooke's Cognitive Examination (MACE, ACE-III) [18, 19];
- or a sentence, as in the Test Your Memory (TYM) test [20].

After a delay period, during which other tests are undertaken in order to prevent the simple verbal rehearsal of the material which is to be remembered, there follows a recall phase. Different tests score the registration and recall phases differently, but for purposes of memory testing it is the delayed recall aspect which is most significant. Memory retrieval may also be probed by the use of cueing (MoCA) or by forced choice between correct and incorrect options (recognition paradigm; ACE-III). Some cognitive screening instruments are recognised to be perfunctory in their testing of memory (e.g. MMSE).

Tests of retrograde memory usually focus on aspects of semantic knowledge such as the names of famous people (e.g. Prime Minister, assassinated US President) or the dates of famous events (e.g. World War I or II). Tests of personal history, recalling memories of significant events from previous decades of the patient's life, are difficult to undertake unless corroboration can be obtained from a reliable family member or friend who knows the patient well. Certainly informant accounts can supplement the clinical assessment of patients with memory complaints, and cognitive screening instruments designed to be completed by informants are available [8].

Factors Affecting Cognitive Assessment

Cognitive screening instruments may be described as "noisy", meaning that factors other than brain pathology may influence patient performance, i.e. the tests may measure things other than what they were designed to measure. Both patient-related and test-related factors may be relevant.

Patient-related factors include age, education, mood state, and sensory impairments. Patient age and educational status are important determinants of test performance, and some cognitive screening instruments attempt to make allowance for patient age (e.g. DemTect) or years of education (e.g. MoCA) in the overall scoring. Normative data allowing correction of MMSE scores to account for patient age and educational level are available but seldom applied in clinical practice. Many cognitive screening test items are heavily dependent on language, and hence are subject to possible educational and cultural biases which present additional challenges to individuals with limited education or from cultures using a different language. Screening tests may need adaptation for these factors, and also for patient ethnicity. Ideally, culture-free cognitive screening tests should be developed. Patient assessment by means of informant reports may be relatively culture-free, as may also be the case for functional assessments.

Primary psychiatric disorders such as anxiety and depression may impact on patient test performance, for example because of agitation and inattentiveness or lack of effort. Qualitative judgments by the test administrator as to how the patient performed the test may need to be taken into account, as well as the overall test score.

In addition to mood state, patient fatigue may also impact performance, although this is less of an issue when using brief cognitive screening instruments compared to the extensive test batteries often used in formal neuropsychological assessment which may take hours to perform [2–4].

The presence of primary sensory deficits, such as visual or hearing impairment, also requires notice since these deficits may impact on the ability to carry out test items which are dependent on these sensory modalities. There is an interrelationship between acquired visual or hearing loss and cognitive impairment, and test adaptations are required to allow for these deficits [21]. At minimum, it should be ensured that if the patient regularly uses eye glasses or a hearing aid these should be available when cognitive testing is undertaken.

Test-related factors include sensitivity, avoidance of floor and ceiling effects and of practice effects. Tests should be sufficiently sensitive to detect cognitive disorders. A test which is insufficiently sensitive will miss possible cases, hence false negatives, whereas a test which is too sensitive will label some normals as cases, hence false positives. When defining appropriate test cut-offs, particular weight may be given to those test accuracy studies which have been conducted in circumstances akin to those in which it is planned that the test will be used, such as day-to-day clinical practice ("pragmatic" studies) [22].

Ceiling and floor effects are best avoided for optimum test utility. Ceiling effect is associated with tests which are too easy, such that many patients score highly or at maximum, in which case they may be erroneously labelled as normal (false negatives). Conversely, floor effect describes tests which are too hard such that many normals score poorly and may be erroneously labelled as cases (false positives). If longitudinal cognitive testing is to be undertaken, floor and ceiling effects make it difficult to observe any change, respectively any worsening or improvement since test scores are already approximating to minimum or maximum.

Practice effects describe the improvement in patient performance if the same test is repeated within a short period of time due to increased familiarity with the test contents. Clearly, for longitudinal monitoring of cognitive function to be meaningful such practice effects should be avoided, for example by having variant forms of tests or ensuring the time between repetitions is sufficient to minimise the risk of practice effects [11]. If not taken into account, practice effects may give a false impression of cognitive improvement.

Aside from these test-related factors which may influence test performance, another shortcoming or criticism which may be levelled at cognitive screening instruments is their ecological or functional relevance. How often in our day to day lives are we required, for example, to subtract 7 s from 100 serially, or to fold pieces of paper in half and place them on the floor (both tests from the MMSE), and are there significant functional consequences if we cannot? Scales specifically assessing function, as opposed to cognition, are available, such as the Instrumental Activities of Daily Living (IADL) Scale, although its ability to screen adequately for dementia may be questionable [23]. The Free-Cog scale, currently in development, is an attempt to incorporate assessment of cognition and function in a single instrument (Prof A Burns, personal communication, February 2017). Combining cognitive and functional scales may facilitate dementia diagnosis [24].

Assessing Postoperative Cognitive Dysfunction

These various considerations regarding patient and test factors which affect meaningful cognitive assessment feed into the study of cognitive dysfunction which occurs following surgical procedures under anaesthesia. Surgery may "unmask" pre-existing but clinically undeclared neurodegenerative disease giving the impression of "acute onset" [25], or may on occasion be associated with the inadvertent damage of memory eloquent structures within the brain [26]. However, these scenarios are unusual, unlike the subtle and long-lasting deterioration in cognitive function seen in some patients which Moller and colleagues have designated as postoperative cognitive dysfunction (POCD) [27, 28]. This is distinct from early postoperative cognitive dysfunction and delirium which are not infrequent sequelae of major surgery in the elderly, perhaps related to residual effects of analgesia and hypnotic medications, pain, and sleep disturbance. POCD is said to be the most common cerebral complication after non-cardiac surgery in elderly patients. The pathogenesis of POCD is uncertain; possible contributing factors include increasing patient age, intraoperative hypoxaemia, arterial hypotension, metabolic-endocrine stress response, and long-acting sedative use.

POCD is defined on the basis of test results; it is detectable only with the use of neuropsychological testing and hence its definition is always open to question depending on which test(s) have been used [29, 30]. Diagnosis of POCD requires comparison of baseline, preoperative, performance on cognitive testing with repeat testing in the postoperative period. Hence this may be seen as equivalent to screening cognitive function in the surgical population.

Recommendations for the assessment of suspected POCD have been published [30], many of which will be familiar from the foregoing discussion about cognitive testing and the limitations of cognitive assessment. These include, *inter alia*:

- Tests should be based on proven sensitivity to detect subtle cognitive dysfunction, test-retest reliability, culture insensitivity, and ease of bedside administration.
- Tests should be suitable for use in surgical patients, with degree of difficulty aimed to minimise floor and ceiling effects.
- Practice/learning effects should be minimised.

Selection of appropriate timing of baseline testing is important, with 1–2 weeks prior to surgery suggested as optimal, to avoid the inevitable anxiety on day of admission. Timing of follow-up assessment also needs consideration, since in the immediate postoperative period issues such as pain, medication, and sleep disturbance may affect test performance.

Repeated test use requires more than one test version to avoid practice effects. In addition, testing of a suitable normative population (age- and ability-matched) at the same time intervals is recommended to allow correction for practice effects and variability between sessions.

The International Study of Post-operative Cognitive Dysfunction (ISPOCD) group has suggested a test battery for detection of POCD.[31] Whether any of the commonly used cognitive screening instruments, rather than this extensive test battery, would be suitable for the detection of syndromes of postoperative cognitive dysfunction has not, to my knowledge, been examined as yet, although in the ISPOCD recommendations MMSE was used as an initial screen, with patients scoring below 24/30 excluded from further assessment [30].

Conclusion

"Cognitive function" describes a spectrum of mental faculties with broad neuroanatomical substrates. Hence the assessment of cognitive function is potentially challenging. A structured approach based upon testing various cognitive domains is required to capture any focal deficits which, if subtle, might otherwise go relatively unnoticed. Formal neuropsychological assessment using extensive test batteries is impractical for routine use, so forms of cognitive screening using relatively simple instruments is a logical first step to determine which patients require more in-depth assessment. The chosen assessment schedule should be selected according to the patient population to be studied (population-based, primary or secondary care, patients undergoing surgical procedures).

Acknowledgement   Thanks to Dr. Lauren Fratalia for critical comments on this manuscript.

References

1. Hodges JR. *Cognitive assessment for clinicians*. 3rd ed. Oxford: Oxford University Press; 2018.
2. Lezak MD, Howieson DB, Bigler ED, Tranel D. Neuropsychological assessment. 5th ed. New York: Oxford University Press; 2012.
3. Mitrushina M, Boone KB, Razani J, D'Elia LF. Handbook of normative data for neuropsychological assessment. 2nd ed. Oxford: Oxford University Press; 2005.
4. Strauss E, Sherman EMS, Spreen O. A compendium of neuropsychological tests: administration, norms, and commentary. 3rd ed. New York: Oxford University Press; 2006.

5. Larner AJ. *Neuropsychological neurology. In: The neurocognitive impairments of neurological disorders* (2nd ed). Cambridge: Cambridge University Press; 2013. p. 1–22.
6. Burns A, Lawlor B, Craig S. Assessment scales in old age psychiatry. 2nd ed. London: Martin Dunitz; 2004.
7. Tate RL. A compendium of tests, scales, and questionnaires. The practitioner's guide to measuring outcomes after acquired brain impairment. Hove: Psychology Press; 2010. p. 91–270.
8. Larner AJ, editor. Cognitive screening instruments. A practical approach. 2nd ed. London: Springer; 2017.
9. Malloy PF, Cummings JL, Coffey CE, et al. Cognitive screening instruments in neuropsychiatry: a report of the Committee on Research of the American Neuropsychiatric Association. *J Neuropsychiatry Clin Neurosci*. 1997;9:189–97.
10. Larner AJ. Introduction to cognitive screening instruments: rationale and desiderata. In: Larner AJ, editor. Cognitive screening instruments. A practical approach. 2nd ed. London: Springer; 2017. p. 3–13.
11. Heilbronner RL, Sweet JJ, Attaix DK, Krull KR, Henry GK, Hart RP. Official position of the American Academy of Clinical Neuropsychology on serial neuropsychological assessment: the utility and challenges of repeat test administrations in clinical and forensic contexts. Clin Neuropsychol. 2010;24:1267–78.
12. Stein J, Luppa M, Brähler E, König HH, Riedel-Heller SG. The assessment of changes in cognitive functioning: reliable change indices for neuropsychological instruments in the elderly – a systematic review. Dement Geriatr Cogn Disord. 2010;29:275–86.
13. Folstein MF, Folstein SE, McHugh PR. "Mini-mental state." A practical method for grading the cognitive state of patients for the clinician. *J Psychiatr Res*. 1975;12:189–98.
14. Nasreddine ZS, Phillips NA, Bédirian V, et al. The Montreal cognitive assessment, MoCA: a brief screening tool for mild cognitive impairment. *J Am Geriatr Soc*. 2005;53:695–9.
15. Kalbe E, Kessler J, Calabrese P, et al. DemTect: a new, sensitive cognitive screening test to support the diagnosis of mild cognitive impairment and early dementia. Int J Geriatr Psychiatry. 2004;19:136–43.
16. Hodkinson HM. Evaluation of a mental test score for assessment of mental impairment in the elderly. Age Ageing. 1972;1:233–8.
17. Brooke P, Bullock R. Validation of a 6 item cognitive impairment test with a view to primary care usage. Int J Geriatr Psychiatry. 1999;14:936–40.

60 A. Larner

18. Hsieh S, McGrory S, Leslie F, et al. The Mini-Addenbrooke's Cognitive Examination: a new assessment tool for dementia. *Dement Geriatr Cogn Disord.* 2015;39:1–11.

19. Hsieh S, Schubert S, Hoon C, Mioshi E, Hodges JR. Validation of the Addenbrooke's Cognitive Examination III in frontotemporal dementia and Alzheimer's disease. *Dement Geriatr Cogn Disord.* 2013;36:242–50.

20. Brown J, Pengas G, Dawson K, Brown LA, Clatworthy P. Self administered cognitive screening test (TYM) for detection of Alzheimer's disease: cross sectional study. BMJ. 2009;338:b2030.

21. Pye A, Charalambous A, Leroi I, Thodhi C, Dawes P. Screening tools for the identification of dementia for adults with age-related acquired hearing or vision impairment: a scoping review. Int Psychogeriatr. 2017;29:1771–84.

22. Larner AJ. Diagnostic test accuracy studies in dementia. A pragmatic approach. London: Springer; 2015.

23. Hancock P, Larner AJ. The diagnosis of dementia: diagnostic accuracy of an instrument measuring activities of daily living in a clinic-based population. Dement Geriatr Cogn Disord. 2007;23:133–9.

24. Larner AJ, Hancock P. Does combining cognitive and functional scales facilitate the diagnosis of dementia? Int J Geriatr Psychiatry. 2012;27:547–8.

25. Larner AJ. "Dementia unmasked": atypical, acute aphasic, presentations of neurodegenerative dementing disease. Clin Neurol Neurosurg. 2005;108:8–10.

26. Ibrahim I, Young CA, Larner AJ. Fornix damage from solitary subependymal giant cell astrocytoma causing postoperative amnesic syndrome. Br J Hosp Med. 2009;70:478–9.

27. Moller JT, Cluitmans P, Rasmussen LS, et al. Long-term postoperative cognitive dysfunction in the elderly ISPOCD1 study. ISPOCD investigators. International Study of Post-operative Cognitive Dysfunction. *Lancet.* 1998;351:857–61. [Erratum: *Lancet* 1998;351:1742].

28. Moller JT. Postoperative cognitive decline: the extent of the problem. Eur J Anaesthesiol. 1998;15:765–7.

29. Rasmussen LS, Moller JT. Central nervous system dysfunction after anesthesia in the geriatric patient. Anesthesiol Clin North Am. 2000;18:59–70.

30. Rasmussen LS, Larsen K, Houx P, et al. The assessment of postoperative cognitive function. Acta Anaesthesiol Scand. 2001;45:275–89.

Chapter 5
Management of Delirium on the Surgical Ward

Shane O'Hanlon

Introduction

Delirium is common on the surgical ward and there are many unique factors that contribute to it in this setting. Traditionally it has not been addressed by surgical teams, with a request for consultation from geriatric medicine or psychiatry teams being triggered on discovery of acute confusion. This chapter describes the changing environment of the surgical ward as the diagnosis and management of delirium has become democratised. Greater awareness of the problem and the effectiveness of getting everyone involved in delirium management has occurred. A new paradigm for addressing delirium on the surgical ward has been established and can be replicated in any surgical ward.

S. O'Hanlon
St Vincent's University Hospital, and University College Dublin, Dublin, Ireland
e-mail: shaneohanlon@svhg.ie

© Springer International Publishing AG, part of Springer Nature 2018
A. Severn (ed.), *Cognitive Changes after Surgery in Clinical Practice*, In Clinical Practice,
https://doi.org/10.1007/978-3-319-75723-0_5

Significance

Delirium is common among surgical patients. In one review of older patients on a surgical ward by de Castro [1], the incidence of delirium was 16.9% (23.2% for acute admission, $P < .001$). Median length of hospital stay was 13 days (range 3–85) for patients with delirium versus 7 (range 1–54) for patients without ($P = .002$).

The occurrence of delirium after surgery is associated not only with an increased risk for prolonged hospital length of stay (relative risk [RR], 1.9; 95% CI, 1.4–2.7), but also a 50% increased risk of discharge to an institution rather than home (RR, 1.5; 95% CI, 1.3–1.7), and an over two-fold increased risk of 30-day readmission (RR, 2.3; 95% CI, 1.4–3.7) [2]. In the same study delirium was found to exert the strongest risk on adverse outcomes at a population level.

The co-occurrence of delirium with cardiac, respiratory, or renal complications was associated with a potentiation of adverse outcomes such as prolonged length of stay (RR, 3.4; 95% CI, 2.3–4.8), discharge to an institution rather than home (RR, 1.8; 95% CI, 1.4–2.5), and 30-day readmission (RR, 3.0; 95% CI, 1.3–6.8). Delirium was a greater potentiator for these adverse outcomes than traditional surgical complications such as returns to the operating room, wound infection, myocardial events, and sepsis. Delirium is also associated with

---

Box 5.1 Common causes of delirium on the surgical ward

Dehydration secondary to bowel obstruction
Post-operative hypoxia
Post-operative pneumonia
Pain related to surgical conditions
Wound or intra-abdominal infections
Electrolyte abnormalities related to ileostomy or fistula
Fast atrial fibrillation related to above problems

long-term mortality [3]. Even one episode of delirium between admission and day three in hospital carries a risk for unanticipated ICU admission or in hospital death [4].

Hazards on the Surgical Ward

In surgical patients a different approach to delirium is necessary. Box 5.1 lists some common causes of delirium in the surgical ward setting. The general physician will be accustomed to seeing quite a different list of causes on the medical ward. Of note is that fact that opiate toxicity is not listed; this much-feared condition occurs very rarely. In fact many surgical patients do not receive regular pain assessment after their care is transferred from the anaesthetic team to the surgical team. This potentially results in poor pain control, something that in itself can precipitate delirium. Use of a tool such as the Abbey pain scale can also help to monitor response to analgesia in patients with cognitive impairment [5]. Side effects of opiates can however contribute to delirium, in particular constipation and urinary retention. Pain can also contribute to behavioural changes in patients with dementia, and it is interesting to note that in a nursing home setting the systematic use of regular analgesia was associated with less agitation [6]. The same principle can be considered in the post-operative setting.

Fluid management is a very commonly misjudged practice among older patients on the surgical ward. Volume status and hydration is difficult to assess – and may be left to the least experienced member of the medical team. Unfortunately it is very common for intravenous fluids to be prescribed without any estimation of fluid and electrolyte requirements. The presence of bowel obstruction or fistulae can further complicate fluid balance and senior review should be provided regularly.

Another factor that complicates fluid prescription is deciding whether older patients have cardiac dysfunction. Easily detected signs such as cardiomegaly on chest x-ray, and raised jugular venous pressure are often missed or ignored. Conversely the presence of peripheral oedema is almost uniformly considered to be a sign of heart failure, when many other factors may be contributing. In unwell surgical patients, hypoalbuminaemia is common and when seen in conjunction with poor mobility can cause significant leg oedema, even in the presence of perfectly normal cardiac function.

Problems with Our Current Approach

Delirium is often missed, and rates of unrecognised delirium still remain around 60% [7]. Characteristically, the patient will have been seen by several healthcare professionals before it is noticed. This happens particularly when the subtype is hypoactive, where the patient may be very quiet and does not seem to warrant much attention compared to the agitated type where everyone on the ward is aware. As a result, the hypoactive type has a poorer prognosis and can last for longer periods.

Delirium is also not emphasised – staff sometimes casually mention that they observe subtle changes in behaviour. These are the valuable observations (often made by care staff) that are minimised, yet should prompt an urgent medical review. It is worth listening to the views of staff who may be close to the patient, doing tasks such as bathing and feeding: their observations about subtle changes in behaviour, e.g. 'not quite herself' or 'seemed a bit off' may be valuable predictors of a looming crisis. A culture change is needed so that if anyone notices something amiss cognitively, at any stage, this is escalated to the appropriate team.

Falls are strongly related to delirium, and there have been calls to introduce delirium prevention quality metrics in an effort to help improve falls rates [8]. Rates of postoperative delirium varied 8.5-fold across hospitals in one study [9], which suggests that some centres have more success than others. This variation in care quality needs to be eradicated.

A New Approach to Delirium

Delirium prevention and management should be led from the hospital boardroom and needs to be emphasised across specialities [10]. Everybody that works in the hospital setting should have mandatory delirium training – this can be practically achieved by embedding it within dementia training. It is important not only for clinical staff, but also for those who do not have regular direct patient contact, as widespread knowledge is needed. This also includes those in management, and there is a strong argument for using electronic records to flag patients with delirium as this can help to predict adverse events and prolonged length of stay.

Prevention

Despite good evidence that delirium rates can be lowered by implementing preventive measures, they have not been widely adopted. A multidisciplinary approach is necessary and it is likely that non-pharmacological approaches are most successful. Because delirium can be caused by multiple triggers, it is necessary to use a multi-component programme. Most of the measures simply involve sensible patient care, e.g. early mobilisation, adequate nutrition and hydration, avoidance of constipation, optimisation of pain control, ensuring rest at night-time, and ensuring visual or hearing aids have been provided if used at home.

The impact of such multi-component interventions can be impressive. One study in the elective setting reported rates of delirium of 16.7% in the control group and 0% in the intervention group, although numbers were small [11]. In a subsequent meta-analysis, a relative reduction of 30% in delirium rates was seen [12]. As well as this benefit, a greater than 60% odds reduction in falls was found with multicomponent interventions in another review [13].

The concept of pharmacological prophylaxis against delirium has been investigated using several agents, without much success. Dexmedetomidine has been proposed as a possible neuroprotective agent to prevent delirium. Liu conducted a randomised trial and showed lower rates of post-op delirium among older patients with mild cognitive impairment undergoing elective hip surgery [14]. However the study involved small numbers, and it is possible that any benefit seen was due to sedation rather than prevention of delirium.

Screening

Since we are poor at picking up delirium, the sensible solution is to screen for it. Early detection can certainly help to modify the course, so there is logic to this approach. There are several tools that one can choose (e.g. the 4AT – weblink https://www.the4at.com/), but all that really matters is that a nominated tool is used widely. In practice, this tends to be especially important where the usual "delirium professionals" such as geriatricians or old age psychiatrists are not seeing patients on a regular basis, or where staff are inexperienced.

Some health professionals will protest that "there is no time for delirium screening" or "there is so much else to do" but the answer to this must be that nothing is more important than preventing delirium. By doing so, one will likely reduce a patient's length of stay and adverse events, improve their quality of life and help to investigate whether they have underlying cognitive impairment.

Another really useful question to ask patients is "Have you seen anything or heard anything that wasn't really there?" It is frequently surprising how many people will answer in the affirmative after a stay in the Intensive Care Unit. This is sometimes made even worse by lodging the patient in a side room on their own. Remember that this is the closest thing to solitary confinement that we can legally do and that we have normalised this medical behaviour!

Risk Stratification

Advanced age is often said to be a risk factor for delirium, but it should not in itself prompt concern. Many 90 year olds will sail through the perioperative period without any cognitive dysfunction, but some 50 year olds with other risk factors will have severe delirium. Advanced age is ultimately just a correlation with increasing comorbidity. Even younger people can get delirium. How is it that a pregnant 30 year old can become delirious when an 80 year old with sepsis may not? The simple way to think of this is in terms of two combining entities:

1. Cognitive reserve
2. Magnitude of the insult

In graphic terms, the better your reserve the stronger the insult needed to trigger delirium. Pre-existing cognitive impairment is the single most important reason that people are at risk of delirium. Those with more advanced dementia are more prone. For such people with low cognitive reserve, delirium may be precipitated by relatively innocuous things such as constipation, mild dehydration or even a ward move. For people who have good reserve it is important to take delirium especially seriously – it signifies that the insult is major and thus needs rapid management. An example would be hypoxia – even a 30 year old will become confused if the oxygen saturation is low enough. It is those patients whom one doesn't expect to become delirious that one needs to worry most about. These patients have a worse outcome than those that are frail (frailty is the gradual accumulation of deficits as individuals age, which results in loss of physiological reserve) [15]. In people with good cognitive reserve who become delirious, they are very unwell and a detailed search for a cause should ensue, with a handover to staff that this process should continue if not concluded by the end of a shift.

Estimating the delirium risk for patients admitted has two advantages. First, it allows high risk patients to be monitored closely so that intervention can occur earlier. Secondly, it permits estimation of the severity of the insult that triggers it. In a person who becomes delirious despite low estimated risk, clinical suspicion should be high for a serious illness. In this case, it means that clinicians should act quickly to rule out a very serious precipitant such as intra-abdominal sepsis.

Happily several precipitants of delirium are easily treated: hypoxia, constipation, infection and others will often respond well to the usual management. If this helps delirium to resolve then one can be reassured that the correct approach has been taken.

The Process of Diagnosis

Delirium diagnosis needs to be democratised – the most junior members of the team should be not only permitted, but encouraged, to make the diagnosis. The easy opt out of "acute confusion" when written in the notes should mean that brief targeted education is directed towards the author. Within the hospital environment there are usually "newer" staff who are open to the importance of delirium, and the more well-established group that may not place any importance on it. After all, it has not been afforded much attention during their career so why change now? This approach should be challenged, and dissemination of the multidisciplinary multicomponent approach should be undertaken.

Multidisciplinary Approach to Delirium Management

Once a patient is recognised to be "high risk of delirium" then a tailored care plan should be put in place. Angel described a standardised approach to management of delirium on medical and surgical units [16]. All of the measures described above in the section on prevention also form the basis of management of delirium. They are equally effective on surgical units as medical wards [17]. By far the most important thing is to identify what is the most likely reason for delirium to have been triggered. This is rarely simply due to surgery itself, and it is more common that there is another particular cause.

Box 5.2 shows the factors necessary for successful management of delirium. Multicomponent interventions such as this are associated with a lower 30 day readmission rate [18].

Patient Management

There are several very practical measures that can be taken when dealing with a delirious patient. First, bed moves should be avoided as they can worsen confusion. In modern hospital settings, it is often the case that a patient will have moved at least three times within their first 48 h of admission. This must be minimised where possible. Regular reorientation is also vital: many of us assume that patients have been well informed of their management plan and also have the cognitive ability to remember that information. In fact it is quite common for people to have no idea where they are, or why they are there several days into a hospital admission. This may not mean they haven't been informed, but rather that delirium has made it impossible for them to process and retain that information. A good approach is to regularly remind people of where they are, what day it is, what time it is, what is happening in their day, and why they are still in hospital. The lack of understanding of why one is in hospital can be very distressing and it is easy to understand how this can lead to agitation or the feeling that you are being kept in against your wishes. These principles of clear communication are extremely important. Much reassurance can be provided by simply helping confused patients to know what is happening.

Symptomatic Control

Many sources will refer to control of symptoms as part of the management of delirium. Great caution should be exercised with this approach as it may prompt omission of thorough investigations to find the cause. There is absolutely no point in using haloperidol to "manage" behavioural disturbance if the reason the patient is confused is their hypoxia. Similarly, if a delirious patient is extremely anxious and trying to get out of bed, but nobody has actually explained where they are and what is happening, then calling the doctor to prescribe lorazepam is only making the situation worse.

Many of these so-called treatments for delirium have the potential for considerable harm and adverse events. The evidence does not suggest that there is a clear benefit to using them [19]. First line measures should always be to build up a clear picture of why the patient is delirious then to put in place an individualised plan to manage the cause and reduce the likelihood of other precipitants. This should particularly be done for patients who clearly have a high risk of developing delirium. Any use of antipsychotic medications should be reviewed every day including at weekends, and the dose weaned at the earliest possible point. If delirium appears to be resolving, then it is appropriate to reduce the dose; but staff should be advised that as delirium fluctuates it may be necessary to maintain availability of a contingency dose in case of exacerbation.

Rehabilitation During and After Delirium

Delirium increases length of stay and part of the reason for this is likely to be the delay in starting rehabilitation in patients that need it. It is not uncommon that several days of rehabilitation are lost as patients with delirium typically lack the attention and focus needed to cooperate with therapy. This compounds the effect of the delirium itself, as the longer older people stay in bed the longer the rehabilitation period they will require.

Close collaboration is required with the MDT so that they can monitor the situation and as soon as the patient is able to participate with rehabilitation they can engage with staff. It should also be noted that experienced rehabilitation staff are in an ideal position to identify patients with delirium as they notice those patients who are disoriented or lack attention. Delirium is associated with a gap in functional recovery at 1 month that never resolves out to the 18-month follow-up [20].

Ward Design

Modern hospitals are often designed with many side rooms, however they should be avoided for delirious patients in many cases. Side rooms are a convenient place in which to dump "troublesome" patients, including those with delirium. This well meaning approach (from the point of other patients) is counterproductive. As mentioned above, being isolated can exacerbate or promote delirium. Nobody, least of all those at risk of or suffering from delirium, should be in a single room without mental stimulation. Patients sometimes linger alone in a room without any meaningful engagement, sometimes not even being aware there is a television. Radio shows, music, newspapers, magazines or puzzles can also help, and patients should be asked if they have a hobby such as craft work or art. Visitors should be encouraged to bring in photos, which have the dual advantage of reorientating patients and making staff realise that they are treating a real person, with an identity, a life and a family that care for them.

Ward Team

Delirium requires a real team effort to recognise and manage it. Everyone has a valid observation, whether health professional, catering staff or porter. For this reason it is essential that regular training sessions are provided and an education board for delirium is also recommended. This can also help family members to read more about the condition to understand how it is identified and managed, and helps to reassure them that the team is taking it seriously.

While the suspicion of delirium is one for which everyone is equipped, the detailed management, once initial surgical causes have been addressed does require the input of specialists who see every patient who has post-operative "confusion". An ideal approach would be an integrated geriatric team that sees all new admissions with the surgical team. This allows rapid screening for delirium, frailty and acute illness. A more thorough comprehensive geriatric assessment can then be undertaken after this brief ward round. Daily geriatrician input is required, but this can be provided mainly by a specialist registrar with consultant support and supervision when needed.

Consent process

Do you mention the possibility of delirium or post-operative cognitive dysfunction? You should! Who else will? Anaesthetists are very well placed to speak about such a significant adverse event related to surgery, unless you have access to a pre-operative geriatrician review. Tomlinson notes that delirium should be considered an integral part of a preoperative discussion of risk, as it is an increasingly well-recognised complication with potentially devastating consequences [21].

Delirium has only recently been recognised in the literature (and not yet in clinical practice) as a postoperative complication [22]. Since it occurs more commonly than many adverse events usually mentioned in the consent process it deserves to be mentioned. In high risk patients it also makes sense that the possibility of not returning to baseline is also outlined. This helps to better inform patients and families about the risks of surgery and to plan for possible increased care needs.

Post-traumatic Stress

None of us should ever underestimate the effect that delirium can have on a person's psychological state. Many patients become visibly anxious when asked to recall their delirium, such is the profoundly disturbing effect it can have. Some centres offer psychological support to help patients to work through this. Patients should be asked if they remain burdened with the distress that delirium can precipitate as they recover. Hallucinations in particular can remain frightening, even several weeks after the symptoms have resolved.

Follow up

Delirium is likely to be a marker of a vulnerable brain [23]. For this reason it marks a sentinel event in a patient's life and should merit further cognitive assessment once recovery has occurred. Full recovery is not always achievable, and in fact delirium can cause permanent cognitive changes. One study showed the close association between an occurrence of delirium and the likelihood of subsequent dementia. During a 5-year follow up period after cardiac surgery, 26.3% of patients developed dementia. Postoperative delirium had occurred in 87% of those who later developed dementia [24].

Delirium in the presence of the pathologic processes of dementia is associated with accelerated cognitive decline beyond that expected for delirium or dementia alone [25]. Patients have linear trajectories of cognitive decline over postoperative months 2–36, and these trajectories were significantly steeper among participants in one study who developed delirium compared to those who did not [26]. In addition, worse cognitive function prior to surgery is significantly associated with faster cognitive decline over follow-up [27]. Given its significance, delirium should prompt the person responsible for the discharge of the patient to ensure that follow up is made at a local specialist memory clinic several weeks after discharge. Even in persons without dementia, cortical atrophy is associated with postoperative delirium severity [28].

Conclusion

Delirium on the surgical ward can be well treated and managed by using multi-component interventions in a multidisciplinary team setting. A hospital wide awareness of the significance of delirium is required. Surgical patients should be evaluated for their delirium risk pre-operatively and screened for its presence in the post-operative phase. Ward design and staffing should be tailored to the needs of this group of patients, whose outcomes can be very poor if the condition is not well managed.

Box 5.2 Factors necessary for appropriate management of delirium in hospital

Hospital management
>   Boardroom support for delirium programme
>   High level medical and nursing knowledge of significance of delirium
>   Funding support for perioperative geriatrician input

Ward level
>   Surgical team support for geriatric input and awareness of need to proactively detect and manage delirium
>   Nursing team skilled in management of delirious patients
>   Physiotherapist who has experience providing encouragement to patients with delirium, who may fear getting out of bed
>   Occupational therapist review available, for assessment of care needs and cognition, or need for adaptations or supportive equipment

Non-medical staff who know to support people with
delirium, e.g. help with eating/drinking, reassurance and
reorientation
Bladder scanner available 24/7

Environment
Well-lit during daylight hours, with low light and noise
levels to support sleep at night
Clear display of time and date
Open visiting without restriction for family of patients
with delirium
Television, radio or reading material provided and
encouraged
Familiar objects such as photos of close family/friends,
blankets

Support & aids
Glasses, hearing aids, dentures provided for patient use
Call bell and drink within reach
Mobility aids individualised for patient needs
Appropriate seating provided

Nursing
Avoid changes in location while delirious– nurse
patient in high dependency area with high staffing ratio
Close monitoring of fluid input and outputs
Offer fluids and snacks regularly
Bowel chart kept accurately
Daily encouragement to sit out or mobilise if possible,
in between physiotherapy input
Encouragement to use own clothes rather than pyjamas
Regular prompts to medical team to remove
intravenous lines, catheter, drains, other tubes
Alert medical team if signs of infection, new or
changing oxygen requirements, constipation, poor
urinary output
Keep low threshold for identification of "confusion" or
disorientation and request medical review when present
Assess care needs regularly and offer help where
appropriate

(continued)

Box 5.2 (continued)

Keep sleep chart and encourage sleep when appropriate to establish regular routine

Medical

Use screening tools to proactively detect delirium

Ensure adequate fluid intake, use intravenous fluids if necessary but stop as soon as adequate oral intake

Review medications for inappropriate prescriptions

Screen daily for post-operative infections

Obtain collateral history of any previous confusion or disorientation

If delirium present, proactively ask if any hallucinations occurring and offer treatment if so

Communication

Use regular introduction – establish a "Hellomynameis" culture

Inform patient and family of diagnosis of delirium

Provide regular reassurance that it is likely to improve once the cause is identified

Ensure all staff aware of diagnosis of delirium

Pre-empt all investigations, blood tests, x-rays etc. with full explanation of rationale

Follow up

Refer to memory clinic when delirium occurs in patient with no prior cognitive dysfunction

References

1. de Castro SM, Ünlü Ç, Tuynman JB, Honig A, van Wagensveld BA, Steller EP, et al. Incidence and risk factors of delirium in the elderly general surgical patient. Am J Surg. 2014;208(1):26–32. https://doi.org/10.1016/j.amjsurg.2013.12.029. Epub 2014 Mar 26
2. Gleason LJ, Schmitt EM, Kosar CM, et al. Effect of delirium and other major complications on outcomes after elective surgery in older adults. JAMA Surg. 2015;150(12):1134–40.

3. Falsini G, Grotti S, Porto I, Toccafondi G, Fraticelli A, Angioli P, et al. Long-term prognostic value of delirium in elderly patients with acute cardiac diseases admitted to two cardiac intensive care units: a prospective study (DELIRIUM CORDIS). Eur Heart J: Acute Cardiovascular Care. 2017. https://doi.org/10.1177/2048872617695235.

4. Hshieh TT, Yue J, Oh E, Puelle M, Dowal S, Travison T, et al. Effectiveness of multicomponent nonpharmacological delirium interventions a meta-analysis. JAMA Intern Med. 2015;175(4): 512–20. https://doi.org/10.1001/jamainternmed.2014.7779.

5. Abbey J, Piller N, De Bellis A, Esterman A, Parker D, Giles L, et al. The Abbey pain scale: a 1-minute numerical indicator for people with end-stage dementia. Int J Palliat Nurs. 2004;10(1):6–13.

6. Husebo BS, Ballard C, Sandvik R, Nilsen OB, Aarsland D. Efficacy of treating pain to reduce behavioural disturbances in residents of nursing homes with dementia: cluster randomised clinical trial. BMJ. 2011;343:d4065. https://doi.org/10.1136/bmj.d4065.

7. de la Cruz M, Fan J, Yennu S, Tanco K, Shin S, Wu J, et al. The frequency of missed delirium in patients referred to palliative care in a comprehensive cancer center. Support Care Cancer. 2015;23(8):2427–33.

8. Lee EA, Gibbs NE, Fahey L, Whiffen TL. Making hospitals safer for older adults: updating quality metrics by understanding hospital-acquired delirium and its link to falls. Perm J. 2013;17(4):32–6.

9. Berian JR, Zhou L, Russell MM, Hornor MA, Cohen ME, Finlayson E, et al. Postoperative delirium as a target for surgical quality improvement. Ann Surg. 2017.

10. O'Hanlon S, O'Regan N, MacLullich AMJ, Cullen W, Dunne C, Exton C, et al. Improving delirium care through early intervention: from bench to bedside to boardroom. J Neurol Neurosurg Psychiatry. 2014;85:207–13.

11. Chen CC, Lin MT, Tien YW, Yen CJ, Huang GH, Inouye SK. Modified hospital elder life program: effects on abdominal surgery patients. J Am Coll Surg. 2011;213:245–52.

12. Martinez F, Tobar C, Hill N. Preventing delirium: should non-pharmacological, multicomponent interventions be used? A systematic review and meta-analysis of the literature. Age Ageing. 2015;44(2):196–204.

13. Hsieh SJ, Madahar P, Hope AA, Zapata J, Gong MN. Clinical deterioration in older adults with delirium during early hospitalisation: a prospective cohort study. BMJ Open. 2015;5(9):e007496. https://doi.org/10.1136/bmjopen-2014-007496.

14. Liu Y, Ma L, Gao M, Guo W, Ma Y. Dexmedetomidine reduces postoperative delirium after joint replacement in elderly patients with mild cognitive impairment. Aging Clin Exp Res. 2016;28(4):729–36.

15. Dani M, Owen LH, Jackson TA, Rockwood K, Sampson EL, Davis D. Delirium, frailty and mortality: interactions in a prospective study of hospitalized older people. J Gerontol A Biol Sci Med Sci. 2017;73:415–8. https://doi.org/10.1093/gerona/glx214.

16. Angel C, Brooks K, Fourie J. Standardizing Management of Adults with delirium hospitalized on medical-surgical units. Permanente J. 2016;20(4):27–32. https://doi.org/10.7812/TPP/16-002.

17. Siddiqi N, Harrison JK, Clegg A, Teale EA, Young J, Taylor J, et al. Interventions for preventing delirium in hospitalised non-ICU patients. Cochrane Database Syst Rev. 2016;3:CD005563. https://doi.org/10.1002/14651858.CD005563.pub3.

18. Rubin FH, Bellon J, Bilderback A, Urda K, Inouye SK. Effect of the hospital elder life program on risk of 30-day readmission. J Am Geriatr Soc. 2017;66:145–9. https://doi.org/10.1111/jgs.15132.

19. Neufeld KJ, Yue J, Robinson TN, Inouye SK, Needham DM. Antipsychotic medication for prevention and treatment of delirium in hospitalized adults: a systematic review and meta-analysis. J Am Geriatr Soc. 2016;64(4):705–14.

20. Hshieh TT, Saczynski J, Gou Y, Marcantonio ER, Jones RN, Cooper Z, et al. Delirium delays functional recovery following elective surgery. Innovation Aging. 2017;1:1326. https://doi.org/10.1093/geroni/igx004.4860

21. Tomlinson JH, Partridge JSL. Preoperative discussion with patients about delirium risk: are we doing enough? Periop Med. 2016;5(1):22. https://doi.org/10.1186/s13741-016-0047-y.

22. Zenilman ME. Delirium an important postoperative complication. JAMA. 2017;317(1):77–8. https://doi.org/10.1001/jama.2016.18174.

23. Fong TG, Davis D, Growdon ME, Albuquerque A, Inouye SK. The Interface of delirium and dementia in older persons. Lancet Neurol. 2015;14:823–32.

24. Lingehall HC, Smulter NS, Lindahl E, Lindkvist M, Engström KG, Gustafson YG, et al. Preoperative cognitive performance and postoperative delirium are independently associated with future dementia in older people who have undergone cardiac surgery: a longitudinal cohort study*. Crit Care Med. 2017;45(8):1295–303.
25. Davis DHJ, Muniz-Terrera G, Keage HAD, Stephan BCM, Fleming J, Ince PG, et al. Association of Delirium with Cognitive Decline in late life a Neuropathologic study of 3 population-based cohort studies. JAMA Psychiat. 2017;74(3):244–51. https://doi.org/10.1001/jamapsychiatry.2016.3423.
26. Inouye SK, Marcantonio ER, Kosar CM, Tommet D, Schmitt EM, Travison TG, et al. The short-term and long-term relationship between delirium and cognitive trajectory in older surgical patients. Alzheimers Dement. 2016;12:766–75. https://doi.org/10.1016/j.jalz.2016.03.005.
27. Devore EE, Fong TG, Marcantonio ER, Schmitt EM, Travison TG, Jones RN, et al. Prediction of long-term cognitive decline following postoperative delirium in older adults. J Gerontol A Biol Sci Med Sci. 2017;72(12):1697–702.
28. Racine AM, Fong TG, Travison TG, Jones RN, Gou Y, Vasunilashorn SM, et al. Alzheimer's-related cortical atrophy is associated with postoperative delirium severity in persons without dementia. Neurobiol Aging. 2017;59:55–63. https://doi.org/10.1016/j.neurobiolaging.2017.07.010.

Chapter 6
Critical Illness and Delirium

Valerie Page and Tamas Bakonyi

Background

Delirium is a clinical syndrome that is caused by acute brain dysfunction, often called acute confusion. In critical illness it is associated with worse outcomes, regardless of age, including long-term cognitive impairment equivalent to moderate traumatic brain injury or mild Alzheimers, increased length of hospital stay and costs [1–3]. The longer the patient has delirium the worse the outcomes.

Prevalence

Critically ill patients have the highest risk of developing delirium due to multiple risk factors linked with their presenting illness, co-morbidities and admission to a critical care

V. Page (✉)
Anaesthesia and Critical Care, Watford General Hospital, Watford, UK

Imperial College, London, UK
e-mail: Valerie.page@whht.nhs.uk, v.page@imperial.ac.uk

T. Bakonyi
Intensive Care, St Mary's Hospital, London, UK

© Springer International Publishing AG, part of Springer Nature 2018
A. Severn (ed.), *Cognitive Changes after Surgery in Clinical Practice*, In Clinical Practice,
https://doi.org/10.1007/978-3-319-75723-0_6

unit itself [4]. The prevalence of delirium in patients in critical care is reported to be up to 74% in critically ill patients with a high severity of illness and approximately 50% in patients who require mechanical ventilation for over 48 hours. Delirium will persist as long as the precipitating causes continue, usually infection or drugs. Because delirium is so common and has such an adverse impact on key outcomes it is essential that critical care clinicians take it seriously, diagnose it, manage the causes and reduce the risk factors.

Pathophysiology

The pathophysiology of delirium is not fully established. There are a number of theories including neuroinflammation, oxidative stress, cerebral hypoperfusion/hypoxia, neuroendocrine abnormalities, neurotransmitter dysregulation, network disconnectivity, circadian rhythm disruption/melatonin dysregulation and aging [5]. These theories are complementary, rather than competing, with many overlapping areas and reciprocal influence.

Whatever the cause of delirium there are a number of core symptoms that fluctuate – inattention, hypo/hyperalert, sleep/wake disturbance. The final common pathway theory, postulated in 2000, suggests that while the appearance of some symptoms may depend on the cause(s), a final common neural disruption is likely to be responsible for core symptoms. Evidence supports a central cholinergic deficiency and associated dopamine excess. Both acetylcholine and dopamine pathways overlap significantly, dopamine (with serotonin and norepinephrine) mediate responses to stimuli modulated by a cholinergic pathway play a key role in arousal. In addition oxidative stress leads to significant increases in dopamine [6].

This neurotransmitter imbalance has been the main target for pharmacological interventions to date. The evidence from brain imaging suggests delirium results in ultimate cerebral atrophy (Fig. 6.1) [7].

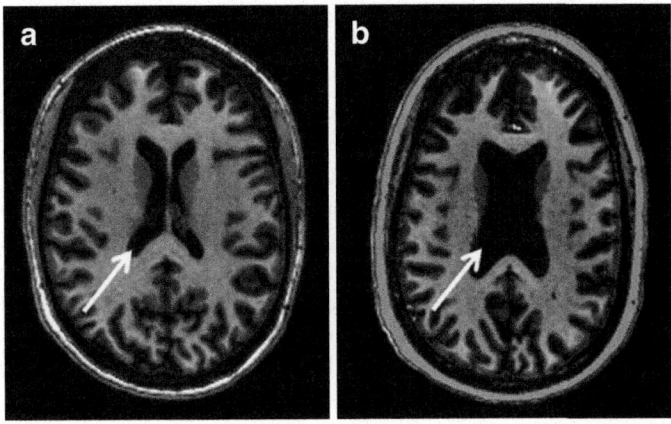

FIGURE 6.1 Representative example of lateral ventricle size in 46-year-old female and 42-year-old female ICU survivors with no preexisting cognitive impairment. Axial T_1-weighted brain images in 2 ICU survivors. (a) Depicts relatively normal ventricular volume (see arrow) in a 46-year-old female who did not experience delirium in the ICU. Patient had a history of respiratory and heart failure. She was admitted to a medical ICU due to acute respiratory distress syndrome (ARDS) and was subsequently intubated and managed through the ICU without ever developing delirium. (b) Depicts enlarged ventricles (see arrow) in a 42-year-old female who did develop delirium in the ICU. Patient was admitted to the hospital after reporting fever and dyspnea with a chest X-ray and other laboratory data confirming community acquired pneumonia and ARDS. The patient was admitted to the ICU and mechanically ventilated, experiencing 12 days of delirium and then resolution. There was no preexisting history of neurological impairment, and surrogate questioning for preexisting cognitive impairment was also negative (Gunther et al. [7])

Motoric Subtypes

Delirium is classified according to the presenting psychomotor activity of the patient, hypoactive, hyperactive and mixed [8]. The most common presentation in critically ill patients is as hypoactive delirium in which the patient is quiet, lethargic and apparently compliant [9]. As a result delirium recognition

is a particular challenge for critical care healthcare professionals. It varies in severity; at its worse these hypoactive
delirious patients show minimal responses to verbal stimulation and are incapable of engaging with standardized testing
or even interview. Hyperactive delirium is easily recognised;
these patients are often combative, insomniac and clearly hal-
lucinating. This form, however, is less common, present in
from 5% up to 22% of ICU patients with delirium [10]. With
the mixed presentation the patient symptoms vary from day
to day or within a day between lethargy to agitation, but
always with inattention, a core diagnostic feature. If clinicians
do not routinely screen for delirium using a validated assessment tool they are likely to miss it and so fail to manage take
steps to manage it.

Recognition

Clinicians can screen for delirium in intubated and ventilated
patients who are on or off sedation, using one of two currently
validated tools the Confusion Assessment Method-ICU
(CAM-ICU) or the Intensive Care Delirium Screening
Checklist (ICDSC) [11, 12]. Further information and resources
to implement either of these assessment tools are freely
available to download from www.icudelirium.org. Patients who
are more deeply sedated cannot be assessed for delirium.

CAM-ICU

The CAM-ICU can be undertaken on any patients who open
their eyes for more than 10 s to a verbal stimulus, such as
responding to their name and takes roughly 2 min to undertake. It assesses four items, delirium can be ruled out at stages
1, 2 or 4 (Table 6.1):
    By contrast the ICDSC does not require the cooperation
of the patient.

TABLE 6.1 The CAM-ICU tool

1. Recognition of change in mental status
   Yes, proceed to 2. No change = no delirium, stop assessment.
2. Inattention – Is the patient able to squeeze the assessors hand on the 'A's in a sequence of letters?
   Yes = no delirium, stop assessment. If not (more than 2 errors) proceed to 3.
3. Level of consciousness other than awake and aware.
   Yes = delirium, stop assessment. No proceed to 4
4. Disorganized thinking – Four yes/no questions and a simple command.
   Fails (more than one mistake) = delirium. Passes = no delirium.

For a demonstration see www.youtube.com/watch?v=6WyJ0zL7VkI

TABLE 6.2 The ICDSC tool	
	Level of consciousness
	Inattention
	Disorientation
	Hallucination/delusion/psychosis
	Psychomotor agitation or retardation
	Inappropriate speech or mood
	Sleep/wake disturbance
	Fluctuation of symptoms

The ICDSC has eight items of which the presence of four is required to establish a diagnosis of delirium (Table 6.2):

The information can be gathered over the course of several hours and so can be incorporated into a single shift of the clinician's time.

The CAM-ICU and ICDSC are validated to be used in all critically ill patients. In around 10% of sedated intubated patients the CAM-ICU will be normal once the effect of sedation wears off [13].

In patients who do not require tracheal intubation or in patients who have been extubated an additional more sensitive assessment of inattention can be used such as spelling the word 'lunch' backwards or saying the months of the year backwards [14, 15]. A patient without inattention, a core feature of delirium, will complete these assessments without mistakes.

Current Advances

There is an increasing interest in the use of EEG in the diagnosis of delirium, the classic changes being described as an increased delta and reduced alpha2 activity [16]. Recently van der Kooi have developed an EEG based tool in non-sedated patients [17]. In patients following cardiothoracic surgery they observed that the relative delta power using two electrodes in a frontal-parietal derivation can distinguish the patients who had delirium from those who did not (Fig. 6.2).

Researchers have developed a test to objectively detect inattention in ICU patients who are awake enough to maintain eye contact for 10 s, which is implemented on a custom-built computerized device. The Edinburgh Delirium Test Box-ICU has potential additional value in longitudinally tracking attentional deficits because it provides a range of scores and is sensitive to change [18].

Management

Treat Cause

Once it is recognised a critically ill patient is delirious or that delirium is continuing the priority is to determine and treat any precipitating cause, there is often more than one. It is vital that any drivers of the delirium are removed or at least reduced as far as possible. In the critical care environment the most common causes of delirium are infection and drugs.

Hence it is important to look for infection, also review electrolyte levels, blood gas analysis, glucose levels, and level

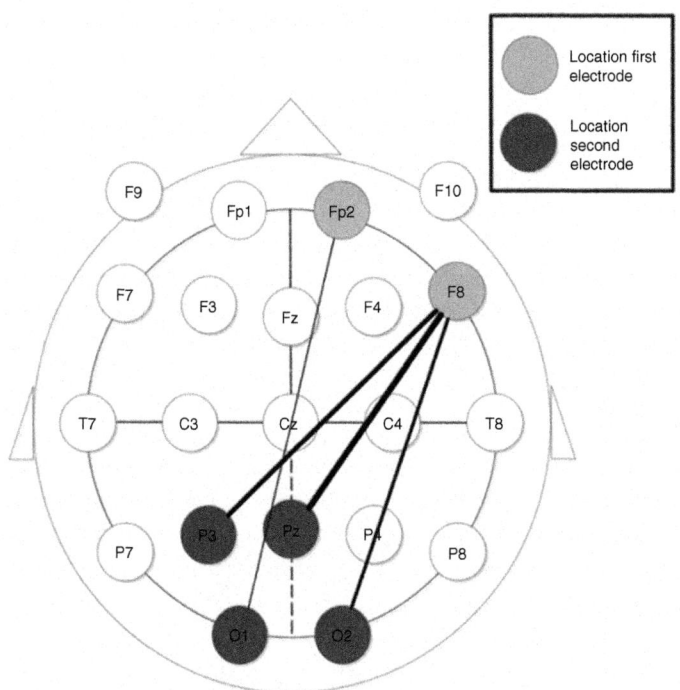

FIGURE 6.2 Delirium detection using EEG – ScienceDirect [17]

of vitamins such as vitamin B12, folate, and thiamine; consider the possibility of toxins or illicit drugs; and assess kidney, liver and thyroid function. All medications must be reviewed regularly and deliriogenic drugs e.g. with anticholinergic activity reduced or stopped if possible [19].

Non Pharmacological Management

Physical Care

Non-pharmacological management of delirium is directed at reducing the modifiable risk factors. The effectiveness of multicomponent preventative bundles on medical and surgical wards is discussed elsewhere in this book – currently there is no evidence that these measures work in critically ill patients but the principles of good practice can be extrapolated from what has been shown to work elsewhere. In the intensive care environment this means that a bundle of holistic and excellent clinical care should promote normal brain and physical function [20]. Essentially the bundle aims to promote normal brain and physical function. This includes regular reorientation of the patient, being able to see a digital clock, facilitating a good night's sleep, providing eye glasses and hearing aids where needed, avoiding constipation or dehydration, and removing any attached monitors, cannulae and tubes as soon as they are not needed. Early mobilisation is essential and has been demonstrated to reduce delirium and accelerate recovery [21]. Mobilising the patient, from passive range-of-motion exercise through to walking will increase cholinergic activity, thought to be imbalanced in delirium. As a minimum patients need to be sat out of bed as soon as it can be done safely.

Sedative Drug Burden

In the ICU drugs are a major risk factor to precipitate or maintain delirium. Critically ill patients who require mechanical ventilation usually require infusions of sedative and analgesic drugs, with the aim they are pain-free and comfortable, with an endotracheal tube in place, when clinical and personal care is given and for effective ventilatory support. These drugs have been implicated in delirium: sedation goal directed protocols need be used in all intubated patients. National and regional evidence-based recommendations are that critically ill patients who require mechanical ventilation are kept awake or lightly sedated, unless deeper sedation is clinically indicated [4, 22–25]. Only a minority of patients will require deep sedation. It has been recommended by an expert group that ideally, the patient be awake in order to maintain eye contact, interact with caregivers and family members and participate in physical and/or occupational therapy but permitted to drift off to sleep when uninterrupted [26].

The Challenge

Only a minority of patients will require deep sedation, however sedation delivery is a complex health care intervention
and the majority of UK critically ill patients who require
mechanical ventilation are kept over sedated. There are a
number of identified barriers including the absence of knowledge of sedation algorithms, insufficient understanding as to
the adverse effects of deep sedation and concern about
patient's well-being and comfort [27–29]. There is an assumption that more nursing staff would be needed to safely keep
patients attached to life-saving devices awake or easily
aroused. There are well-documented issues relating to communication between doctors and nurses, a lack of direction by
medical staff and not having the means to manage an agitated
or lightly sedated patient. Nurses describe a lack of support,
a limited understanding of the indications and impact, and
consistently concerns around patient agitation. All of these
issues need to be addressed at a local level if a daily sedation
target is to be achieved in the majority of patients.

A standard daily sedation goal protocol will generally
include:

- Providing good analgesia, usually alfentanil, fentanyl or
  remifentanil by infusion with additional fentanyl or morphine boluses for nursing interventions as required
- Effective management of agitation: reassurance, reorientation and if needed an antipsychotic for delirium or a
  small dose of propofol or benzodiazepine for fear or
  anxiety.
- Low dose infusion of sedative infusion, commonly propofol, rate adjusted as needed for general comfort.

The Drugs

Benzodiazepines are a known risk factor for delirium and are
best avoided unless patient or staff safety is at risk in severe
agitation, anxiety or the patient is suffering alcohol withdrawal. Bolus administration is preferred because of the risk

of cumulation of long acting drugs given by infusion [30]. In the UK propofol infusions are used in the majority of patients and are associated with more favorable outcomes than midazolam [31].

The alpha2-agonists, dexmedetomidine and clonidine, achieve sedation via a different receptor-mediated pathway. They have less effect on respiratory function, possess analgesic effects and it has been suggested dexmedetomidine may allow better patient communication [32, 33]. One study using it in intubated delirious agitated patients showed a reduction in delirium by approximately a day as compared with placebo in 72 patients [34]. Dexmedetomidine is expensive compared to other agents and licensed for ICU use. In contrast, clonidine is very cheap and while unlicensed for sedation is widely used in the UK for management of agitation, as an intravenous bolus or an infusion [35].

Other Drugs

Many of the drugs given to critically ill patients have anticholinergic properties; this includes metoclopramide, ranitidine, theophylline, furosemide, digoxin, and analgesics (although pain is also a risk factor for delirium). https://www.drugs.com/article/anticholinergic-drugs-elderly.html#drug-list   Given that reduced cerebral acetylcholine has been hypothesized to be the common final pathway in the development of delirium in response to inflammation, anticholinergic drugs are biologically plausible as a risk factor in delirium. While a relationship between drugs with anticholinergic properties and delirium has not been demonstrated, taking into account the altered drug handling in critical illness it is good clinical practice to review all medications with a view to stopping any not needed [36].

The data regarding steroids and delirium is inconclusive, one large trial observed an increase in risk of delirium in critically ill patients, another did not [37]. A single-centre substudy within the Dexamethasone for Cardiac Surgery

(DECS) trial showed no difference in delirium outcomes in the ICU patients randomized to dexamethasone or placebo [38]. One recent controlled study found that hydrocortisone use in patients with sepsis reduced the incidence of delirium although there were some issues regarding number of delirium assessments [39]. Currently there is insufficient evidence to support steroid use as a cause for delirium or as a therapy to reduce delirium. Given other side effects the wise clinician would reserve the use of steroids for an evidence based indication.

Pharmacological Treatment

There are no drugs to date which have been proven to reduce delirium in critically ill patients although drugs may be useful to manage agitated symptoms either as a sole therapy or as an adjunct to sedative drugs. The first drug of choice in managing agitation as a result of delirium is an antipsychotic.

Haloperidol

Haloperidol is a butyrophenone, its main action is as a dopamine antagonist. It is the only antipsychotic that can be administered intravenously and it is the most used and studied antipsychotic drug for ICU delirium prevention and treatment. It remains the most commonly used and useful drug in the UK, although it is not now licensed for intravenous use [40]. A double-blind randomised controlled trial showed haloperidol, as compared with placebo, did not decrease delirium in critically ill patients, however haloperidol treated patients were less agitated [41]. Haloperidol is contraindicated in patients with prolonged QTc because of a potential risk of torsades de pointes, a dangerous ventricular arrhythmia and ECG monitoring is needed. It is also contraindicated in Parkinson's disease and can rarely cause neuroleptic malignant syndrome. It is extensively metabolised in the liver.

Neuroleptic malignant syndrome is a rare but potentially fatal side effect. It is usually diagnosed clinically; the patient classically develops symptoms of rigidity, high temperature and autonomic dysregulation [42]. Blood tests will show an elevated creatine phosphokinase levels and leucocytosis. It can lead to permanent neurological impairment with survivors left with parkinsonism and cognitive impairment. The treatment of neuroleptic malignant syndrome is mainly supportive; it is directed toward controlling the rigidity and hyperthermia and preventing complications (e.g., respiratory failure, renal failure). The use of dantrolene is controversial.

Haloperidol is usually given as a slow intravenous bolus, if the enteral route can be used then an antipsychotic with less side effects such as quetiapine or risperidone would be preferable. Current clinical practice is to use an initial dose of 2.5–5 mg, wait 30 min and repeat if needed. For end of life care it can be used subcutaneously and mixed in the same syringe as an opioid and an antiemetic if needed.

Atypical Antipsychotics

The term 'atypical' has been used for those antipsychotic drugs manufactured after the 1990s. They bind more loosely to dopamine receptors than haloperidol, dissociate more readily and demonstrate a high level of serotonin occupancy. Olanzapine is the only other antipsychotic that can be given parenterally, and it is given by intramuscular injection. It is useful for when symptoms need managing in a patient where enteral medication is not an option, haloperidol is contraindicated or in units that do not use haloperidol following the removal of its license for intravenous use. The National Institute of Clinical Excellence (NICE) guidelines suggest the use of olanzapine, for the short-term management of distress (NICE, 2010) [43]. The US Pain, Agitation, and Delirium guidelines concluded that there is limited evidence for the use of atypical antipsychotics.

Alternatives to olanzapine are quetiapine and risperidone, the evidence to date does not support their use to prevent or treat delirium. A recent trial in palliative care showed distressing behavioural, communication, and perceptual symptoms of delirium were significantly greater in those treated with antipsychotics (risperidone or haloperidol) than in those receiving placebo [44].

Anti-cholinesterases and Anti-inflammatory Drugs

Given the final common pathway theory of delirium, an excess dopamine and a relative hypocholinergic state, rivastigmine, an anti-cholinesterase drug, was hypothesised as a useful treatment for ICU delirium. However a multi-centre trial was stopped early at 104 of a planned 440 patients because there appeared to be a signal for harm with increased mortality in the rivastigmine group and increased duration of delirium. It is not recommended for use in critically ill patients [45].

Simvastatin by virtue of its anti-inflammatory properties was investigated in mechanically ventilated patients but was shown not to decrease days of brain dysfunction – coma or delirium- as compared to placebo in ventilated patients [46]. It may be, however, that patients already on statin medication are at risk of delirium if it is stopped in critical care [47]. Statin medication needs to be continued if possible bearing in mind the patient's liver function and interactions with other drugs e.g. amiodarone and macrolide antibiotics.

Other Considerations

Patient and Family

Talking to the families of critically ill patients about delirium and providing them with information is important. Family members and close friends find witnessing delirium in a loved one extremely distressing. There is an information leaflet free to download at www.icusteps.org the website of the intensive care patient support charity ICUsteps.

In many cases the delirious experience includes terrifying hallucinations and patients often remember it in detail. While the delirium is ongoing, it is probably helpful to talk to patients about their delusions and hallucinations, generally by asking "is anything odd going on/happened?". Delirium can be easily mistaken for depression, and it is important not to miss delirium [48]. Once the delirium has cleared, talk to patients openly about delirium and ask them about perceptual disturbances while being sensitive to the fact that some patients would prefer not to talk about their hallucinations at that time. This opportunity to talk about delirium can be repeated in the ICU follow up clinic when survivors often want to talk about and understand about their critical illness experience.

Establishing a direct link between delirium and post-traumatic stress disorder post intensive care in critical care survivors has been investigated but to date a robust link has not been found [49]. Patients who appear distressed or who are depressed, have symptoms of post-traumatic stress disorder or in whom delirium persists when all medical and drug causes have been managed would benefit from referral to a hospital liaison psychiatric service.

Conclusion

Awareness of delirium diagnostic criteria and risk factors will assist with prompt recognition and management, improvement in quality of care and so potentially avoiding long term consequences. When assessing patients healthcare professionals need to remember delirium, reduce the risk and treat the cause. Critical care patients need individualized management of delirium precipitants and supportive strategies. For a video summary of the elderly hospitalised patient: https://www.youtube.com/watch?v=qmMYsVaZ0zo, for additional information and resources: www.icudelirium.org.

References

1. Mehta S, Cook D, Devlin JW, et al. Prevalence, risk factors, and outcomes of delirium in mechanically ventilated adults. Crit Care Med. 2015;43:557–66.
2. Pandharipande PP, Girard TD, Jackson JC, et al. Long-term cognitive impairment after critical illness. N Engl J Med. 2013;369:1306–16.
3. Vasilevskis E, Holtz C, Girard T, et al. The cost of delirium in the intensive care unit: attributable costs of care intensity and mortality [abstract]. J Hosp Med. 2015;10(Suppl 2). Accessed 29 Mar 2017.
4. Barr J, Fraser GL, Puntillo K, et al. American College of Critical Care Medicine. Clinical practice guidelines for the management of pain, agitation, and delirium in adult patients in the intensive care unit. Crit Care Med. 2013;41(1):263–306.
5. Cerejeira J, Nogueira V, Luís P, Vaz-Serra A, Mukaetova-Ladinska EB. The cholinergic system and inflammation: common pathways in delirium pathophysiology. J Am Geriatr Soc. 2012;60:669–75.
6. Trzepacz PT. Is there a final common neural pathway in delirium? Focus on acetylcholine and dopamine. Semin Clin Neuropsychiatry. 2000;5(2):132–48.
7. Gunther ML, Morandi A, Krauskopf E, et al. VISIONS Investigation, VISualizing Icu SurvivOrs Neuroradiological Sequelae. The association between brain volumes, delirium duration, and cognitive outcomes in intensive care unit survivors: the VISIONS cohort magnetic resonance imaging study. Crit Care Med. 2012;40(7):2022–32.
8. Stagno D, Gibson C, Breitbart W. The delirium subtypes: a review of prevalence, phenomenology, pathophysiology, and treatment response. Palliat Support Care. 2004;2:171–9.
9. Peterson JF, Pun BT, Dittus RS, Thomason JW, Jackson JC, Shintani AK, Ely EW. Delirium and its motoric subtypes: a study of 614 critically ill patients. J Am Geriatr Soc. 2006;54:479–84.
10. Boettger S, Nuñez DG, Meyer R, et al. Brief assessment of delirium subtypes: psychometric evaluation of the delirium motor subtype scale (DMSS)-4 in the intensive care setting. Palliat Support Care. 2017;15:535–43.
11. Ely EW, Margolin R, Francis J, et al. Evaluation of delirium in critically ill patients: validation of the confusion assessment

method for the Intensive Care Unit (CAM-ICU). Crit Care Med. 2001;29(7):1370–9.

12. Bergeron N, Dubois MJ, Dumont M, Dial S, Skrobik Y. Intensive care delirium screening checklist: evaluation of a new screening tool. Intensive Care Med. 2001;27(5):859–64.

13. Patel SB, Poston JT, Pohlman A, et al. Rapidly reversible, sedation-related delirium versus persistent delirium in the intensive care unit. Am J Respir Crit Care Med. 2014;189:658–65.

14. Han JH, Wilson A, Vasilevskis EE, et al. Diagnosing delirium in older emergency department patients: validity and reliability of the delirium triage screen and the brief confusion assessment method. Ann Emerg Med. 2013;62(5):457–65.

15. O'Regan N, Ryan DJ, Boland E, et al. Attention! A good bedside test for delirium? J Neurol Neurosurg Psychiatry. 2014;85:1122–31.

16. van der Kooi AW, Slooter AJC. EEG in delirium: increased spectral variability and decreased complexity. Clin Neurophysiol. 2014 Oct;125(10):2137–9.

17. van der Kooi AW, Zaal IJ, Klijn AF, et al. Delirium detection using EEG: what and how to measure. Chest. 2015;147:94–101.

18. Green C, Hendry K, Wilson ES, et al. A novel computerized test for detecting and monitoring visual attentional deficits and delirium in the ICU. Crit Care Med. 2017;45:1224–31.

19. Hein C, Forgues A, Piau A, et al. Impact of polypharmacy on occurrence of delirium in elderly emergency patients. J Am Med Dir Assoc. 2014;15:850.311–5.

20. Siddiqi N, Harrison JK, Clegg A, Teale EA, Young J, Taylor J, Simpkins SA. Interventions for preventing delirium in hospitalised non-ICU patients. Cochrane Database Syst Rev. 2016;(3):CD005563. https://doi.org/10.1002/14651858. CD005563.pub3.

21. Schweickert WD, Pohlman MC, Pohlman AS, et al. Early physical and occupational therapy in mechanically ventilated, critically ill patients: a randomised controlled trial. Lancet. 2009;373:1874–8.

22. Whitehouse T, Snelson C, Grounds M. Intensive Care Society review of best practice for analgesia and sedation in the Critical Care 2014. https://www.ics.ac.uk/ICS/guidelines-and-standards. aspx. Last accessed 11 Sept 2017.

23. Barr J, Fraser GL, Puntillo K, et al. Clinical practice guidelines for the management of pain, agitation, and delirium

in adult patients in the intensive care unit. Crit Care Med. 2013;41(1):263–306.

24. Celis-Rodríguez E, Birchenall C, de la Cal MÁ, et al. Clinical practice guidelines for evidence-based management of sedoan-algesia in critically ill adult patients. Federación Panamericana e Ibérica de Sociedades de Medicina Crítica y Terapia Intensiva. Med Intensiva. 2013;37:519–74.

25. DAS-Taskforce 2015, Baron R, Binder A, et al. Evidence and consensus based guideline for the management of delirium, analgesia and sedation in intensive care medicine. Revision 2015 (DAS-guideline 2015) – short version. Ger Med Sci. 2015;13:Doc19.

26. Vincent JL, Shehabi Y, Walsh TS. Comfort and patient-centred care without excessive sedation: the eCASH concept. Intensive Care Med. 2016;42(6):962–71.

27. Everingham K, Fawcett T, Walsh T. 'Targeting' sedation: the lived experience of the intensive care nurse. J Clin Nurs. 2014;23:694–703.

28. Sneyers B, Laterre P-F, Perreault MM, Wouters D, Spinewine A, et al. Current practices and barriers impairing physicians' and nurses' adherence to analgo-sedation recommendations in the intensive care unit – a national survey. Crit Care. 2014;18:655.

29. Sneyers B, Laterre PF, Bricq E, Perreault MM, Wouters D, Spinewine A. What stops us from following sedation recommen-dations in intensive care unit? A multicentric qualitative study. J Crit Care. 2014;29:291–7.

30. Zaal IJ, Devlin JW, Hazelbag M, et al. Benzodiazepine-associated delirium in critically ill adults. Intensive Care Med. 2015;41:2130–7.

31. Lonardo NW, Mone MC, Nirula R, et al. Propofol is associated with favorable outcomes compared with benzodiazepines in ven-tilated intensive care unit patients. Am J Respir Crit Care Med. 2014s;189:1383–94.

32. Mo Y, Zimmermann AE. Role of dexmedetomidine for the pre-vention and treatment of delirium in intensive care unit patients. Ann Pharmacother. 2013;47:869–76.

33. Jakob SM, Roukonen E, Grounds RM, et al. Dexmedetomidine vs midazolam or Propofol for sedation during prolonged mechanical ventilation two randomized controlled trials. JAMA. 2012;307(11):1151–60.

34. Reade MC, Eastwood GM, Bellomo R, et al. Effect of Dexmedetomidine added to standard care on ventilator-free time in patients with agitated delirium: a randomized clinical trial. JAMA. 2016;315:1460–8.

35. Richards-Belle A, Canter RR, Power GA, et al. National survey and point prevalence study of sedation practice in UK critical care. Crit Care. 2016;20:355.

36. Wolters AE, Zaal IJ, Veldhuijzen DS, et al. Anticholinergic medication use and transition to delirium in critically ill patients: a prospective cohort study. Crit Care Med. 2015;43:1846–52.

37. Schreiber MP, Colantuoni E, Neufeld KJ, Needham DM. Comparing analyses of corticosteroids and transition to delirium in critically ill patients. Intensive Care Med. 2017;43:1933–5.

38. Dieleman JM, Nierich AP, Rosseel PM, et al. Dexamethasone for cardiac surgery study group (2012) intraoperative high-dose dexamethasone for cardiac surgery: a randomized controlled trial. JAMA. 2012;308:1761–7.

39. Keh D, Marx ETG, et al. Effect of hydrocortisone on development of shock among patients with severe SepsisThe HYPRESS randomized clinical. Trial JAMA. 2016;316:1775–85.

40. MacSweeney R, Barber V, Page V, et al. A national survey of the management of delirium in UK intensive care units. QJM. 2010;103:243–51.

41. Page VJ, Ely EW, Gate S, et al. Effect of intravenous haloperidol on the duration of delirium and coma in critically ill patients (Hope-ICU): a randomised, double-blind, placebo-controlled trial. Lancet Respir Med. 2013;1:515–23.

42. Oruch R, Pryme IF, Engelsen BA, Lund A. Neuroleptic malignant syndrome: an easily overlooked neurologic emergency. Neuropsychiatr Dis Treat. 2017;13:161–75.

43. National Institute for Health and Clinical Excellence. Delirium: prevention, diagnosis and management. NICE guideline (CG103). 2010.

44. Agar MR, Lawlor PG, Quinn S, et al. Efficacy of oral risperidone, haloperidol, or placebo for symptoms of delirium among patients in palliative care: a randomized clinical trial. JAMA Intern Med. 2017;177:34–42.

45. van Eijk MM, Roes KC, Honing ML, et al. Effect of rivastigmine as an adjunct to usual care with haloperidol on duration of delirium and mortality in critically ill patients: a multicen-

tre, double-blind, placebo-controlled randomised trial. Lancet. 2010;376:1829–37.

46. Page VJ, Casarin A, Ely EW, et al. Evaluation of early administration of simvastatin in the prevention and treatment of delirium in critically ill patients undergoing mechanical ventilation (MoDUS): a randomised, double-blind, placebo-controlled trial. Lancet Respir Med. 2017;5:727–37.

47. Morandi A, Hughes CG, Thompson JL, et al. Statins and delirium during critical illness: a multicenter, prospective cohort study. Crit Care Med. 2014;42:1899–909.

48. O'Sullivan R, Inouye SK, Meagher D. Delirium and depression: inter-relationship and clinical overlap in elderly people. Lancet Psychiatry. 2014;1:303–11.

49. Svenningsen H. Associations between sedation, delirium and post-traumatic stress disorder and their impact on quality of life and memories following discharge from an intensive care unit. Dan Med J. 2013;60:B4630.

Chapter 7
Legal Aspects of Cognitive Impairment

Gary Rycroft

Before the advancement of modern medical techniques in life saving treatments for palliative care and the extension of life beyond what was seen as "normal" decisions were less complex. We now have "choices" our grandparents did not. As a society, we have medicalised death. Society has moved away from the local community, stepping in at the end of life. Lancaster University holds The Elizabeth Roberts Oral History Archive. It contains interviews carried out in the 1970s with people who were born in the 1880s, 1890s and early 1900s and lived in Preston, Lancaster and Barrow. Clearly, all those people have now died, but what they were born into and recall in the

---

The following Chapter sets out the legal position in the jurisdiction of England and Wales as at 1st March 2018. It should not in any way be construed as bespoke legal advice, but rather is intended as guidance only to the reader.

G. Rycroft
Joseph A. Jones & Co Solicitors LLP, Lancaster, UK
e-mail: Gary.rycroft@jajsolicitors.co.uk,
http://www.jajsolicitors.co.uk

© Springer International Publishing AG, part of Springer Nature 2018
A. Severn (ed.), *Cognitive Changes after Surgery in Clinical Practice*, In Clinical Practice,
https://doi.org/10.1007/978-3-319-75723-0_7

archive is a world before the NHS. In those days, the community looked after each other; people spoke to each other. In the UK we rightly celebrate the NHS but one outcome of the NHS is that as a society we have become reliant on things being done to us rather than doing things for ourselves.

Yet we are living in an era where we also recognise the right of a patient to make decisions, but unless there is some framework in place that anticipates a time when a patient may lose mental capacity then all of the advances made with regard to autonomy and informed consent fall down if there is a lack of capacity. Talking to a patient about treatment options presupposes that the patient concerned has mental capacity and clearly in many acute medical situations that is not the case. Advance Care Planning is a way of bridging the gap in that regard and ensuring that there is in effect a conversation between the doctor and patient even if the patient is lacking capacity at the relevant time. It is dealt with later in this chapter, but first of all let us consider some of the essential elements of how the law deals with the difficult problem of patients with varying degrees of cognitive dysfunction presenting in acute care settings. Hopefully this will equip the clinician with understanding of the legal principles underpinning medical practice in this vulnerable group of patients.

The issue of mental capacity, i.e. the ability of the patient to understand and agree to proposed treatments is dealt with in section 1 of the Mental Capacity Act (MCA) of 2005 The MCA is a legal framework which has at its heart the principle that all persons over 16 are deemed to have mental capacity unless proven otherwise. They are seen to have autonomy and have the right to be consulted on matters of their treatment'. The five principles of the MCA can also be stated thus:

1. An assumption of mental capacity for all persons aged over 16.
2. The need for there to be supported decision making for anyone who may be lacking mental capacity.
3. The recognition that making an unwise decision does not necessarily mean there is a lack of capacity.

4. The need for any decision made on behalf of a person who is lacking capacity to be made in "the best interests" of that person.
5. If a decision is to be made on behalf of someone who is lacking capacity then it should be the least restrictive option available.

The Two Stage Test for Mental Capacity: What Is a Valid Decision?

The MCA also sets out a 'two stage' test with regard to assessing if a person has mental capacity to make a particular decision as follows:

1. Is there an impairment or disturbance in the functioning of the person's mind or brain?
2. Is the impairment or disturbance sufficient that the person lacks capacity to make the decision?

With regard to the second stage of the test, according to Section 3(1) of the MCA person is unable to make a decision if they cannot:

- understand the information about the decision being made;
- retain that information in their minds;
- use or weigh up the information as part of the decision process or communicate their decision (whether verbally or by any other mean).

The process is well explained in non technical language by Farmer [1] in his book "Grandpa on a Skate Board" and an handy acronym for remembering the principles of assessment is the acronym "UR toilet" arising from "understand","retain", "weigh up","communicate".

'Unwise' Decisions

The principle enshrined in the MCA that a patient is legally entitled to make an unwise decision is the touch point of conflict of the MCA with the concept of paternalism. The MCA and in particular the statutory backing for unwise decisions therein is a deliberate departure by Parliament from paternalism and is a bold statement about the right of self-determination. In practice, examples where the right to make an unwise decision can cause real issues are in respect of a patient declining surgery which in so doing puts their life at risk and also the patient who is determined to be discharged home into conditions which those caring for the patient consider to be a risk to the patient. In essence – and crucially in law- an unwise decision is one reached where the person making the decision is able to understand, remember and weigh up a set of facts and communicate a decision about those facts, even though someone else considering the same facts may come to an entirely different – and in the view of others, less risky – decision. Further, if a patient has made an unwise decision at a time they have the mental capacity to do so, that decision should not be ignored at later date if the patient later lacks capacity. In those circumstances, a "best interests" meeting about the patient should always consider the known views of the patient at a time the patient had mental capacity.

Advance Care Planning: The Medical, Social, Ethical and Historical Background

A potential solution to the dilemma faced by clinical staff in making proxy decisions about best interest in patients with limited cognitive ability is the concept of Advance Care Planning (ACP). ACP anticipates the time when a client has lost capacity and so may not actively take part at the relevant time in decisions about their care. ACP is a way of clients sending a message to their future selves and future carers about the type of care they would like to receive.

Advance Care Planning (ACP) anticipates the time when a client has lost capacity and so may not actively take part at the relevant time in decisions about their care. ACP is a way of clients sending a message to their future selves and future carers about the type of care they would like to receive.

As we will see, there are some Caveats to that in that no-one (whether having capacity or not) can demand futile treatment. ACP is **not** about assisted suicide/dying. At the time of writing this Parliament and the Courts have decided that that is not legal.

History has had a part to play in the ethics of Advance Care Planning. Nazi war crimes and particularly atrocities carried out in the name of "medical research" has led to the concept of patient autonomy with regard to medical care. We now very firmly understand and believe that patients should decide for themselves and indeed this has led to the idea of "informed consent".

Here is an extract from Sky News on 27th September 2017:

"Top Judge urges Living Wills for vulnerable, elderly or sick people".

A Senior Judge has suggested people should make "Living Wills" in order to set out their wishes in the event of serious incapacitating illness. High Court Judge Mr Justice Francis who is based in the Family Division suggested there should be a campaign to educate people about Living Wills. He said they would resolve cases where a single elderly person no longer has the physical or mental capacity to make their own decisions. The Judge's comments to lawyers came amid a Court of Protection Hearing about the treatment of an elderly man who is in a minimally conscious state. The Court of Protection considers issues about people who lack the mental capacity to make decisions. Mr Justice Francis said "it should be compulsory that we all have to make Living Wills because these cases would be resolved much more easily. We all ought to be encouraged to tackle these issues. If there was some sort of campaign to educate people about these sorts of things, I think people would actually do something about it." Mr Justice Francis said that man's family had been in "great conflict" with hospital staff over-treatment which had led to "intimidation" and "nurses in tears". He said the case was "very, very sad".

In essence, Advance Care Planning is putting in hand arrangements for a patient to speak at a time when they can no longer speak or communicate a decision because of a lack of mental capacity. It is a 'message in a bottle' that a patient wishes to wash up just at a time when a crucial decision about their future care and/or medical treatment is being made on their behalf. It is a way of a patient having their voice heard. There are different types of Advance Care Planning, some of which are legally binding and others which are not but even if they are not legally binding should be considered to be persuasive on anyone caring for a client in the future and indeed making a "best interests" decision about the patient.

Encouraging a conversation about Advance Care Planning is the first step. Encouraging a patient to talk to their loved ones or their care providers about the type of care they would like to receive in the future will never be a bad thing. Many people simply will not talk about future care. It is a taboo for them and so for them whether they get the care they would like in the future or not is going to be a lottery. In the time honoured phrase "if you don't ask you don't get". Hopefully having a conversation with patients when the opportunity arises will lead on to putting in place Advance Care Planning which has a legal basis.

Advance Care Planning: The Legal Framework – Options

Lasting Power of Attorney for Health and Welfare

Sections 9 to 14 of the MCA expanded the role of a legal document called Lasting Power of Attorney (LPA) and for the first time (2005) made it possible to appoint an Attorney to make decisions about health and welfare. Until the 2005 Act was enacted (ironically it came into force only in 2007) the LPA could be applied only to decisions about financial matters. An LPA regarding health and welfare is drawn up in advance but is activated by the Attorney only when the patient (the Donor) is deemed to be lacking in capacity and cannot be voluntarily activated by the donor in advance of this. It is possible to make reference in the LPA for health and welfare to the Attorneys following a "Letter of Wishes" or some other guidance in addition to the LPA as to how they should carry out their roles. These other documents could take the form of an Advance Decision to Refuse

Treatment or an Advance Statement. If prepared in the appropriate way, an Advance Decision to Refuse Treatment is in itself legally binding. An Advance Statement is not legally binding in itself but clearly has weight in terms of any "best interests" decisions which are made on behalf of the client.

Advance Decision to Refuse Treatment (ADRT)

Sections 24 to 26 of the MCA 2005 set out the requirements for a valid ADRT. An ADRT is a legally binding document which sets out circumstances where a client would want medical treatment to be refused on their behalf. It is legally binding so must be followed by any medical professionals who are caring for the client in the future. If a client has expressly stated that he or she does not want to risk receiving certain medical treatment and in certain circumstances and then treatment is carried out in contravention of those wishes then it would amount to an assault. Clinicians will be aware that, for example, a Jehovah's witness who wishes to avoid having a blood transfusion will sign a consent form specifically scripted to reflect this deeply held conviction. Such a form is *de facto* an ADRT about the particular treatment of blood transfusion and failure to observe this would be assault.

Some points to note about ADRTs as per the legislation:

- ADRTs are for those aged 18 plus only
- A patient must have capacity to make an ADRT
- An ADRT should set out refusal of treatment at a time the patient lacks capacity
- An ADRT may express wishes in layman's terms (but of course the more precise the wording, the less room for interpretation)
- An ADRT should be in writing and witnessed – withdrawal of all or part of an ADRT need not be in writing
- Making an LPA for Health & Welfare automatically revokes an earlier ADRT

Advance Statement

An Advance Statement (AS) is a document which sets out a person's preferences for future care. It is **not** legally binding and can cover any number of issues from the preferred setting of care to things like food and drink preferences and spiritual beliefs. Whilst an Advance Statement is not legally binding, it is clearly of high relevance when a decision is being made about an incapacitated person because with reference to the five principles of the MCA, such a decision has to be in the "best interests" of the patient What is in the "best interests" of a patient is going to be an objective test (is the views of the clinical staff unless there is evidence apparent from the patient which can turn it into a subjective test. The obvious way for a patient to bring his or her own evidence to the arena of a "best interests" decision is by making an Advance Decision.

LPA for Health and Welfare v ADRT

An LPA for Health and Welfare takes precedence over an ADRT in terms of the chronology of the document. Any ADRT made before an LPA for Health and Welfare is deemed not to be valid and so a solution is to make an LPA for Health and Welfare and then re-sign her ADRT afterwards. That way, the LPA for Health and Welfare would come before the ADRT.

Do Not Attempt Cardiopulmnary Resuscitation (DNACPR) Orders

According to the Resuscitation Council (UK), in the UK fewer than 10% of people in whom a resuscitation attempt is made outside hospital survive and the figures are only slightly above that (between 10% and 20%) for people in hospital.

The 2014 Court of Appeal decision in Tracey v Cambridge University Hospital NHS and Others [2] ruled that patients should be consulted in relation to Advance DNACPR decisions save in exceptional circumstances. In other words doctors cannot 'mark' a patient as "DNACPR" without discussing that with the patient first. An Attorney under an LPA for Health and Welfare could make such a decision on behalf of an incapacitated Donor if allowed under the LPA for Health and Welfare (in other words if the Donor has gone for so called "Option A" whereby the Attorneys may make decisions about the refusal of life sustaining treatment).

No-one can demand futile medical treatment and doctors can make it clear that CPR and other medical treatment at the end of life would be futile and so they would not carry it out. The 1993 judgement on Airedale N.H.S. Trust v Bland [3] and a succession of cases involving Jehovah's Witnesses have also upheld the legal right for patients to say 'no' to medical treatment. This, of course, is acceptable for those with the capacity to say 'no'. Those lacking capacity are left in the hands of the doctors unless they have made an LPA for Health and Welfare decisions and have discussed matter with their Attorneys or have a made an LPA for Health and Welfare and have made an ADRT.

Many patients would be surprised to learn that the well-used phrase "next of kin" has no legal basis whatsoever; there is no-one in law who has a right to make decisions about another person's health and wellbeing and the only failsafe way that a patient can ensure that their chosen person makes those decisions is by making an LPA for Health and Welfare.

What safeguards does the surgical team have if making a decision on 'best interests' in a patient who lacks capacity? An LPA and its interpretation by the Attorney named in the LPA may be sufficient, but in cases of doubt there is an additional service upon which a clinician may call.

This is the Independent Mental Capacity Advocacy (IMCA) service which is available on a 24 h basis. Its members, people who act on behalf of patients who lack capacity at the request of clinicians, are not legal professionals but are trained in the interpretation of the Act and its implications.

Clinicians, Capacity and Consent for Surgery

It follows that the process of obtaining informed consent for surgery places the medical team under many obligations when it is considered desirable to operate on a patient who lacks capacity. Decisions on emergency life saving treatment may be made without reference to the mental capacity, but the majority of such decisions do not fall into such a category. Surgery to fix a hip fracture, for example is typically undertaken within a widow of opportunity of 24–48 h, theoretically allowing the surgical team time to establish whether a patient has an existing LPA or ADRT. Planned surgery for, for example, bowel cancer gives the team a longer period of time period. The process by which the team seeks the existence of such a document is described as demonstrating compliance with the Mental Capacity Act. Conversely, a clinician who sought to ignore the patient's wishes as expressed in an ADRT by failing to enquire of its existence could be seen to be acting in contravention of the Act. In practical terms it is sensible for a member of the surgical team to make enquiries about possible LPA or ADRT part of standard admission or preoperative assessment preparation, in the same way that the team might seek information about medical or social history.

It is incumbent on the surgical team to be aware of recent changes in the law that have effectively reduced the ability of the team to make proxy and paternalistic decisions. It is of note that such changes have been recognised in modern medical school curricula.

References

1. Farmer T. Grandpa on a skateboard: the practicalities of assessing mental capacity and unwise decisions. Gorleston, UK: Rethink Press; 2016.
2. R (Tracey) v Cambridge University Hospital NHS Foundation Trust and others [2014] EWCA Civ 822R.
3. *Airedale N.H.S. Trust v Bland* [1993] A.C. 789 House of Lords.

Index

© Springer International Publishing AG, part of Springer   113
Nature 2018
A. Severn (ed.), *Cognitive Changes after Surgery in Clinical
Practice*, In Clinical Practice,
https://doi.org/10.1007/978-3-319-75723-0

The manufacturer's authorised representative in the EU is Springer
Nature Customer Service Centre GmbH, Europaplatz 3, 69115 Heidelberg,
Germany. If you have any concerns regarding our products, please
contact ProductSafety@springernature.com

Printed and bound by CPI Group (UK) Ltd, Croydon, CR0 4YY

23/04/2026

02095602-0001